Pathological correlation after cardiac surgery

Pathological correlation after cardiac surgery

Sally P. Allwork MPhil, PhD

Curator, British Heart Foundation Museum of Heart Disease, Institute of Child Health, Hospital for Sick Children, London; Honorary Lecturer in Cardiac Anatomy and Morphology, Royal Postgraduate Medical School, Hammersmith Hospital, London

Foreword by

Professor M. J. Davies, British Heart Foundation
Cardiovascular Pathology Unit, St George's Hospital
Medical School, London

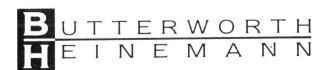

Butterworth–Heinemann Ltd
Halley Court, Jordan Hill, Oxford OX2 8EJ

 PART OF REED INTERNATIONAL P.L.C.

OXFORD LONDON GUILDFORD BOSTON MUNICH NEW DELHI
SINGAPORE SYDNEY TOKYO TORONTO WELLINGTON

First published 1991

© **Butterworth–Heinemann Ltd, 1991**

British Library Cataloguing in Publication Data

Allwork, Sally P.
   Pathological correlation after cardiac surgery.
   1. Coronary diseases. Pathology
   I. Title
   616.120759

ISBN 0-7506-1248-7

Library of Congress Cataloging-in-Publication Data

Allwork, Sally P.
   Pathological correlation after cardiac surgery/Sally P. Allwork.
      p.   cm.
   Includes bibliographical references and index.
   ISBN 0-7506-1248-7 :
   1. Heart–Surgery–Complications and sequelae.   2. Autopsy.
   3. Heart–Pathophysiology.   I. Title.
   [DNLM: 1. Autopsy.   2. Heart Diseases–pathology.   3. Heart
   Diseases–surgery.   W 800 A443p]
   RD598.A45   1991
   617.4'1201–dc20
   DNLM/DLC   90-15172
   for Library of Congress   CIP

Composition by Genesis Typesetting, Laser Quay, Rochester, Kent
Printed and bound by Hartnolls Ltd, Bodmin, Cornwall

Foreword

Audit of the morbidity and mortality of any procedure is an integral part of modern surgical practice; such audit requires the acquisition of accurate data concerning the events. In this context the autopsy, having been in decline, is once again being recognized as an invaluable part of the audit exercise. To provide accurate and pertinent data the pathologist must, however, have considerable knowledge of clinical procedures and practice, and nowhere is this more true than in cardiac surgery. We are in an era when most pathologists have little 'hands on' clinical experience before entering pathology, and unless he happened to train in a centre where specialist cardiac surgery is carried out there is little opportunity to acquire knowledge of the procedures involved. Cardiac surgery for both congenital and acquired disease is now common and many patients live for a considerable time, coming ultimately to autopsy in the District General Hospital or under the Coroner's system. Thus the aquisition of knowledge concerning the long-term effects of cardiac surgery depends on the skills of pathologists not previously exposed to that subject. The answer to this problem lies in the provision of textbooks written by those with both clinical and pathological expertise in the subject. Dr. Sally Allwork is well qualified on both these counts, being closely concerned with the pioneer development of open heart surgery at the Hammersmith Hospital, associated with which she has used her training in anatomy and pathology. The product, a textbook of pathological correlation after cardiac surgery, answers a clear need for any pathologist faced with occasional or regular autopsies on subjects who have undergone cardiac surgery.

It should be considered why such autopsies are difficult. The answer lies in a need for the pathologist to know exactly what the procedure involves and how to define what, if anything, went wrong. Dr. Allwork's text clearly describes the common adult aquired diseases for which surgery is carried out, and explains how to demonstrate whether saphenous vein grafts are patent, and the complications inherent in the myriad types of valve prosthesis which are now used. Unless pathologists clearly record the complications of each type of valve, it may never be known which is best suited to a particular clinical situation.

In the field of congenital heart surgery there are now numerous palliative or corrective procedures, often known by the name of the inventor, such as the Mustard or Fonton procedure. Any meaningful autopsy can be based only on a knowledge of what correction or palliative procedure was attempted. The text by Dr. Allwork provides such knowledge. All these procedures are now allowing subjects to survive into adult life, and it is imperative that data is obtained on the late results and what changes occur, for example in the pulmonary vasculature. In short, a copy of Dr. Allwork's book is a required tool for any pathologist who is going to carry out an autopsy after cardiac surgery, whether this be for a congenital or an acquired condition.

Preface

This book is intended as a guide for those performing necropsies on patients who have at some time undergone a surgical operation on the heart. The operation to bypass coronary lesions is probably the most common surgical operation in the Western world at the present time, so that any pathologist, irrespective of association with a Cardiac Surgical Unit, may be required to perform a necropsy on a sometime surgical patient. Similarly, although surgically treated congenital heart malformations form but a minute proportion of the population, such a patient may 'appear' virtually anywhere. Several years ago such a case was referred to the author, as the appearance of the heart was such that at first sight it was hard to tell which was the anterior and which the posterior aspect! It was this patient (who had had a radical procedure for complete transposition of the great arteries) who stimulated this work.

The author had the good fortune to join the first Cardiothoracic Unit in the UK in 1959, so has been associated with cardiac surgery in general, and with operations utilizing cardiopulmonary bypass in particular, since its infancy. Much of what was learned in the operating room in those early days proved invaluable in later years in the post-mortem room.

The book is not intended to be a treatise on either cardiac surgery or cardiac pathology. It is an account of observations in cardiac surgical necropsies and, as such, is offered in the hope that it may facilitate the task of other prosectors in the interpretation of post-mortem findings, both early and late, after cardiac operations.

Throughout the text 'early deaths' are those which occur within 30 days of the operation; the remainder are all described as 'late deaths'. This follows the convention used worldwide in cardiac surgery with respect to 'early' and 'late' events.

Contents

Part I

Acquired heart disease

1

Post-mortem appearances and routine examination

The body

Almost all operations on the heart using cardiopulmonary bypass (usually called 'open' operations) are done through a midline skin incision and a median sternotomy; there is therefore nearly always a long sternal scar. The thoracotomy is always drained, leaving additional small scars marking the respective positions of the drains. Coronary artery bypass procedures often involve the use of either or both long saphenous veins, so that there may also be long scars on the medial aspect of the legs. Occasionally veins from the arms are used when saphenous veins are unavailable (previous operation) or are unsuitable (varices), and the internal thoracic arteries are increasingly being used as grafts.

Operations in which cardiopulmonary bypass is not used (the so-called 'closed' procedures) are generally performed through a lateral thoracotomy. Most of these are outside the scope of this book, which is concerned with necropsies after open procedures, but some patients have had more than one procedure.

In a few centres, median sternotomy is approached through a submammary skin incision, but as this approach tends to bleed more it is not generally chosen, despite the good cosmetic result.

Operations performed through a *left* thoracotomy include closed mitral valvotomy (now obsolete as a first operation for mitral stenosis, except as an emergency procedure during pregnancy), resection of coarctation of the aorta (irrespective of the technique employed), closure of patent ductus arteriosus, pericardiectomy, and many of the 'shunt' operations to increase circulation to the lungs in congenital malformations causing cyanosis.

Many patients who have had operations to replace the mitral valve have also had closed mitral valvotomy in the more distant past, so that their bodies carry the scar of a left thoracotomy as well as the median sternotomy. Previous median sternotomy is less obvious, as the midline is incised anew. There is no limit to the number of times that median sternotomy may be performed on the same individual.

Right thoracotomy is almost entirely confined to palliative operations for cyanotic congenital heart disease.

As with median sternotomy, drains are invariably laid after lateral thoracotomy. The latter is approached through the bed of the third to the fifth rib and the rib is excised to allow closure of the wound.

Although nowadays the cannulations for bypass (see p. 6) are almost always made directly into the heart and proximal aorta, there are a few occasions on which groin cannulation (the usual technique in the 1950s and early 1960s) is preferred. The conditions in which groin cannulation may still be used are:

1. Reoperation, especially in acute infective endocarditis.
2. Haemorrhage, e.g. from stabbing.
3. Aneurysms of the ascending aorta, particularly if rupture is imminent or has already occurred.

In addition to the surgical wounds there are usually some skin punctures (the sites of venous and arterial lines) and, in early postoperative deaths, there may also be small wounds in the chest wall where pacemaker wires have been removed, either on the ward or in the operating room. (It would be most helpful to the prosector if all of these lines and wires, including the chest drains, could either be left *in situ* or cut short, but apart from the aesthetic sensibilities of those who have the duty to prepare the body for removal, there are some obvious logistical problems, especially where chest drains are concerned.)

Complications

Complications arising from the foregoing procedures are not entirely confined to early postoperative deaths, but *the most common cause of death in the immediate postoperative period is bleeding.*

Haemorrhage

Patients who are Jehovah's Witnesses are obvious risks, but there are others: for example, the elderly (over about 70 years); those undergoing reoperation; those with sepsis; and those taking anticoagulants outside the therapeutic range.

Total exsanguination, in the author's experience, has been confined to Jehovah's Witnesses. In the others the body is pale but with blood in all the cavities. This blood is 'watery' because the cardiopulmonary bypass circuit is primed with watery fluids, not blood. It is usual for the haematocrit to be between 25 and 30% at the end of bypass.

Low cardiac output syndrome

Low cardiac output syndrome is characterized clinically by hypotension, low urine output and cyanosis, despite a normal blood volume. Patients with poor myocardial function may be difficult to wean from bypass and require large amounts of vasopressor agents or circulatory assistance from an intra-aortic balloon pump.

Patients who fail to 'come off bypass', i.e. who are unable to support sufficient arterial pressure to give a cardiac output, do so as a result of poor myocardial function. It is impracticable specifically to evaluate this clinical manifestation at necropsy, but kidney failure in life, with the later finding of acute tubular necrosis, subendocardial necrosis, bowel ischaemia and infarction of the adrenal cortex, together with the finding of cerebral oedema and/or necrosis, are all indicative of death from low cardiac output syndrome.

Intra-aortic balloon counterpulsation

A balloon is introduced into the descending aorta via the femoral artery. It is inflated with carbon dioxide gas to provide counterpulsation and triggered by the electrocardiograph (ECG) to support the cardiac output. Although perhaps more commonly used to support preoperative patients, intra-aortic balloon counterpulsation is sometimes used in the postoperative period as well. At necropsy a fairly common finding is dissection of the femoral artery or fracture of advanced atherosclerotic lesions, with resultant ischaemic damage to the leg. Iatrogenic injury to the aorta is less common, although dissection is possible in aortas with advanced atheroma. Rupture of the balloon may precipitate dissection.

Other complications

Adhesion of the sternum to the underlying structures may damage the specimen irrevocably if considerable care is not taken during removal of the anterior chest wall. This applies particularly to coronary artery operations in which the internal thoracic artery has been used, to patients who have had several operations and in patients who have had conduits placed.

Osteomyelitis of the sternum is a rare complication of median sternotomy, but in elderly patients, especially those with osteoporosis, wound healing may be slow and imperfect.

Chest drains may have been placed accidentally through a coronary artery, the liver, the bowel, the stomach or the thoracic duct. In the case of mediastinal drains, such accidents may result in tamponade or in acute pericarditis. In the case of pleural drains (and the pleural cavity is always drained if it has been entered), haemothorax, pneumothorax or, very uncommonly, chylothorax, may result. Reports in the literature of such mishaps are uncommon but, while rare, do occur. Although more usually causing trouble with drainage in living patients, and therefore treated by revision of the wound, occasionally a drain is caught under a sternal wire.

Swabs may have been left in the chest either accidentally or, more commonly, deliberately. 'Deliberate' swabs are always placed so that they are obvious and are easy to find. Wound swabs are white, all the others are coloured (often green) and all have a radio-opaque marker incorporated into them. The finding of a coloured swab always indicates that it was left by accident.

Several products for procuring haemostasis may be used at operation, and at post-mortem these can at first look very much like swabs. They are quite easy to distinguish from swabs by gentle manipulation: they tend to crumble, whereas swabs remain firm.

Instruments used in the chest are mainly large and long-handled, so that the likelihood of their being lost in the chest is rather remote. However, there is the possibility that a small item, such as a clip, might have escaped the count if the patient died on the table and chest and wound closure were post-mortem procedures.

Venous and arterial lines seldom cause complications. They are usually removed at death without leakage, but occasionally a central venous line, inserted percutaneously into the external jugular vein, causes a local haemorrhage. Because the tubing is of such small gauge, any bleeding resulting from its removal is unlikely to cause significant blood loss in life, but post-mortem leakage can mimic a bleed and thus be rather misleading.

Many surgical patients have temporary *pacing wires* inserted into the anterior wall of the right ventricle. Removal of the wire in the postoperative period, especially if it has to be left for a week or 10 days, is a cause of death from tamponade; part of the thin right ventricle may be removed with the wire. This is a particular risk in chronic sepsis, severe ischaemia and old age.

The heart

Cardiopulmonary bypass

With the rare exception of groin cannulation, mentioned above, all preparations for cardiopulmonary bypass are as follows.

The heart is exposed by longitudinal incision of the pericardium. The right atrium is cannulated, usually through a small incision in the tip of the atrial appendage. A single catheter is generally used for adult patients but bicaval cannulation is necessary in some congenital anomalies. (Use of a single venous catheter tied securely into the atrium means that the patient cannot be perfused by 'total' cardiopulmonary bypass, as only part of the venous return is excluded from the circuit ('partial' bypass). This is usually immaterial to the prosector but operation reports can be misleading and confusing if their writer fails to appreciate this difference, which can be important in living patients.)

The aorta is cannulated through a stab wound, usually made vertically, and controlled by a purse-string suture. The left ventricle is almost invariably vented through a controlled stab incision. Rarely an incision may be made in the left atrium instead and controlled in the same way. All the cannulae are held securely in place by snares.

During bypass the heart is isolated from the perfusion of the rest of the body, both by the venous drainage and by a cross-clamp applied to the aorta proximal to the aortic cannula. The heart itself is protected by cardioplegia, given directly into the aortic root, and sometimes also by coronary perfusion.

At the end of the procedure in adults, the atrial appendage is ligated; in children, it may be closed by suture. The aortotomy is secured by the purse-string and may additionally be buttressed with felt, especially in older patients. The ventricular vent is also secured over a patch of felt.

Examination of the heart

The following techniques are suggested as a routine and a guide; specific points, such as the approach to a particular anomaly and the likely findings, are described with the particular malformation or disease.

First examine the incisions for bypass and the cardiotomy, if present, as their appearance may be helpful in deciding how best to proceed with the rest of the examination; there is often much to be learned early on.

In patients with congenital cardiac malformations it is mandatory to identify the visceroatrial situs and the anatomy and connections of the systemic veins, and to recognize anomalies of pulmonary venous connection, before removing the thoracic contents. The heart and lungs should be retained together; they are also weighed together.

In acquired disease, after excluding pneumothorax (which is extremely rare in the early postoperative period following cardiac surgery because of the invariable practice of chest drainage), care must be taken to ensure that the specimen includes the origin of the left internal thoracic (internal mammary) artery in patients who have had coronary artery bypass operations. As in any other necropsy, dissection of the aorta may be identified before extracting the thoracic contents.

If bleeding from the aortotomy was suspected, it is convenient to make a preliminary examination through a small incision in the pericardium before proceeding. The source can sometimes be identified at this stage.

Pulmonary embolism is very rare in early postoperative death after cardiac surgery, partly because almost without exception the patients are anticoagulated for 4 or 5 days after operation, and partly because they are mobilized on the second or third postoperative day. As with any other patients, those most at risk are patients who may have been immobilized by their illness for a long period awaiting operation, and those with severe varicose veins.

It is convenient in acquired heart disease to separate the heart from the lungs. The pericardium may be examined and removed at the same time. Care should be taken to ensure that all the aortic incisions are retained intact, and that the left atrium is not damaged. Similarly, nicks and lacerations to the heart are to be avoided, especially if it is intended to perform post-mortem coronary arteriography. The heart may be weighed at this stage; it can be reweighed after it has been fixed, opened and washed.

Where possible, only the minimum of dissection should be done before fixing the specimen, as so much is lost if the general morphology is radically modified. Prolonged fixation is unnecessary, as is the use of strong formalin for this purpose. Immersion for 1 or 2 days in 2–5% formalin is adequate for adult hearts, but a few hours suffices for small specimens. The dissection is easier as the tissue is not too hard. Obviously many hearts must be at least partially examined fresh, but transection of the valve rings should be avoided and the caveat about arteriography borne in mind.

Cardiac massage: most deaths in the early postoperative period occur despite intensive resuscitation. Internal massage may produce contusions of the heart and, in extreme cases, disruption of a wound closure or even avulsion of a coronary artery. External massage usually causes contusions of the posterior cardiac surface, and sometimes of the anterior one as well. If there is a mechanical valve *in situ* the cage may cause severe laceration of the left ventricle. Transverse sternal fracture is common, but rib fracture is not. In babies, even in the most skilled hands, there is usually marked contusion of the lungs where they have been compressed by the ribs.

Assessment of the incisions

If there is no obvious gap in the wound (in the case, for example, of a stitch having torn out), the best method is to make a new cut alongside the surgical wound and examine and gently probe from the inside. There may be small tears within (especially in a thin atria and older patients), which permit the passage of the probe and may have leaked but are invisible from the outside.

Sequence of examination

The *right atrium*: whether assessing prosthetic valves or identifying congenital anomalies, the optimal view of the right atrium is gained by opening from the inferior vena cava to the tip (or its remnant) of the right atrial appendage. The venous connections are identified and the atrial septum examined for patency of the foramen ovale.

The *tricuspid valve* should be assessed for morphology and disease (particularly competence or otherwise of the leaflets) before cutting the annulus. The simplest method is to fill the ventricle with water but it is not always easy to assess minor degrees of incompetence in the dead organ. In surgical practice valve sizes are always measured as diameters and prosthetic valves are also sized according to diameter so that it is convenient to have a set of obturators for this purpose.

The *right ventricle* is then opened at the acute margin, incising to the apex and taking note of any aortocoronary bypass graft crossing the acute margin. The incision is continued upwards through the trabecular zone and into the infundibulum, passing to the side of any ventriculotomy. This gives a good exposure of both the walls and the septum.

The *ventricular septum* can now be examined. If a defect, whether congenital or acquired, has been patched, the nature of the patch (e.g. Teflon felt, pericardium;

continuous or interrupted sutures; whether any sutures are torn; whether there are leaks) can be examined. Patches for ischaemic defects of the ventricular septum (VSDs) are irregularly shaped and are often buttressed with felt. Because of ongoing myocardial necrosis they may be 'probe patent'. Patches closing congenital VSDs are regular in shape; they may be applied by either continuous or interrupted suture technique.

The *pulmonary outflow tract* and pulmonary valve may now be examined. Again it may be preferable to measure the diameter of the pulmonary valve rather than its circumference, particularly where the outflow tract is obstructed or has been resected, so that useful correlation may be made with the preoperative investigations and the operation findings.

In congenital anomalies the thickness of the right ventricular wall is measured at the inlet (just below the papillary muscles), at the apex and in the infundibulum. In acquired disease the measurement is made just below the posterior papillary muscle group.

Note the status of the ductus arteriosus or its ligament.

The *left atrium* is best opened obliquely from the right upper pulmonary vein to the tip of the atrial appendage. The reason for this is that, although very rare, there may be a previously undiagnosed 'membrane' between the pulmonary veins and the mitral valve (cor triatriatum sinister) which would otherwise be destroyed.

The pulmonary veins, atrial septum and mitral valve are examined as described for their right-sided counterparts.

The *left ventricle*: test the mitral valve for competence and note its morphology and size before cutting through the ring. In most acquired heart disease it is necessary to transect the apex, usually prior to fixation. As it is desirable to retain the specimen in one piece if possible, this slice and any others should not be completely amputated. Care must be exercised to avoid damaging coronary grafts.

Open the chamber through the obtuse margin of the heart, again noting any grafts. If there is a prosthetic valve in place the ventricle must be incised below it. Continue the incision to the apex, then upwards to the aortic valve, again avoiding or carefully transecting any vein- or arterial grafts traversing the surface. Wall thickness may be measured just below the anterior papillary muscle group. This approach gives good access to the septum and, if the chamber is not grossly hypertrophied, to the aortic root as well.

The *aortic valve* can be measured and then opened, the better to examine the leaflets. Examination of the aortic root is described in Chapter 4 as it is particularly relevant to infective endocarditis.

The *coronary arteries*: if post-mortem coronary arteriography is to be performed it must be done on the unfixed specimen. The coronary arteries are cannulated through the aorta. They may then be rinsed to dislodge post-mortem thrombus, but care must be taken to avoid simultaneously dislodging any ante-mortem thrombus being sought. It is better to use a barium-based medium for post-mortem arteriography as the less viscid, non-ionic contrast media diffuse rapidly into dead tissue and spoil the X-rays. The barium may be mixed with 15% gelatin and formalized with up to 2% by volume of formaldehyde immediately prior to injection to obtain a permanent preparation.

Whether or not they are injected, the coronary arteries are best examined by transverse cuts, close together, along the length of the artery. In postoperative necropsies it is usually unhelpful to open a coronary artery longitudinally as occlusions are thereby destroyed, and dissection of the artery is difficult to assess by this method. The technique does however display the extent of plaque, and grading of the atheromatous disease is facilitated.

The examination of bypass grafts is described in Chapter 5.

The ascending aorta, the arch, isthmus and descending aorta are assessed last.

Complications of cannulation and cardiopulmonary bypass

Placement of the aortic cross-clamp necessitates some dissection, not only between the aorta and the pulmonary artery but also of the epicardial fat between the aorta and the right atrium. This dissection can be a source of troublesome bleeding in life which at necropsy appears as an extensive haematoma; this can make assessment of the incisions difficult.

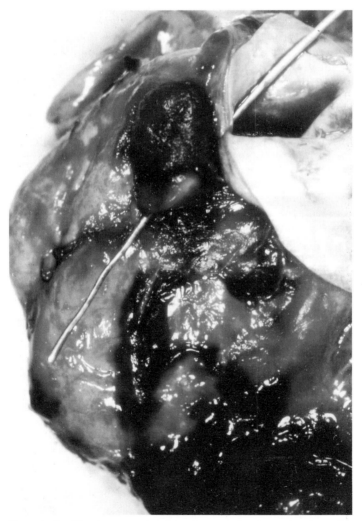

Figure 1.1 Leaking aortotomy 6 months after operation for aortic valve replacement. The probe passes through the small hole which permitted a massive haemopericardium

At operation the aortotomy is often difficult to secure with good haemostasis, particularly in people over about 70 years of age, so that in addition to the blood there may be a relatively large amount of both felt, over the incision itself, and of commercial haemostatic material packed around the aorta. Bleeding from the aortotomy is a cause of death either from exsanguination, because control of haemorrhage from a friable aorta was impossible, or from tamponade, both early in the postoperative period and up to several weeks or even months after operation. As a late event it is more likely in hypertensive patients and those with active endocarditis, but is not confined to them (Figure 1.1).

Haemostatic agents such as gel foam may be mistaken for surgical swabs, but they are easy to identify if it is remembered that haemostatic materials are crumbly in texture, increasingly so as time from operation advances, and are also small. Swab sizes begin at 10×10 cm and increase to anything up to 60×30 cm. Wound swabs are white, while those used for other purposes during the operation are coloured, often green. All swabs have an X-ray detectable thread. White wound swabs are sometimes deliberately left in the field but coloured ones are not, so that their presence deserves comment. The operation note nearly always indicates that a wound swab has been left electively. The usual reason is to try to stop bleeding when all other measures have failed.

In most patients the aortic cannulation site is generally trouble free, probably because the small incision is made vertically, so is less liable to dissect. In elderly patients with less elastic aortas it may be a site of haemorrhage, but the aortotomy is a greater hazard. Although the aortic cross-clamp is, by definition, applied transversely, this site, proximal but close to that of the aortic cannulation, is a rare place for a dissection to begin, although small (up to 1 cm), transverse tears of the intima occur with such frequency as to be unremarkable.

The right atrial appendage is seldom implicated in fatal, early postoperative bleeding but a small, slow leak can in time cause a large haematoma or haemopericardium and may be responsible for late death from tamponade.

The site of the left ventricular vent seldom leaks in the postoperative period as it is usually easy to secure perfect haemostasis at operation. When healing is complete, the felt supporting the purse-string is macroscopically indistinguishable from the native tissues, but the appearance of the apex of the left ventricle is abnormal. The apex appears to be very thin, even in patients with no history of infarction or ischaemia. If transillumination is applied, the apex is translucent.

Microscopically the felt is covered with scar tissue and the surrounding area is fibrotic. (In living postoperative patients the appearance at ventriculography may mimic the apical dyskinesia seen in ischaemic heart disease, so that one may be asked to exclude this, even in young people.)

The leg incisions present no complications peculiar to cardiopulmonary bypass.

2

Materials and prostheses

All materials used inside the heart are 'permanent' in that they are non-absorbable. Contemporary suture materials are of man-made fibres and may be of single thickness (monofilament), stranded or braided. Several types of fabric are used; they may be non-woven (felt), woven or knitted from synthetic yarns. Some of the woven cloths are manufactured as a cylinder and these are often crimped in a tight concertina fashion to allow greater freedom of movement for arterial grafts. Most of these have an X-ray detectable strip woven into them and many of the graft materials unravel when they are cut, necessitating care when examining them at necropsy. Most of the commonly encountered materials are perhaps more widely known by their registered trade names rather than their composition: for example, Teflon felt and two-way-stretch Dacron for patching, and crimped Dacron and Gore-Tex for grafts. Plastics are used to make parts of artificial valves and some prosthetic devices for annuloplasty.

In addition to the man-made products, there are several natural materials which are used in cardiac surgery. These may be taken from the patient at the operation (autologous tissue), from another human being (homologous) or from another species (heterologous or xenograft). Autologous tissues include saphenous veins, pericardium, pulmonary valve, and (now obsolete) fascia lata. Homologous tissues include aortic valves, pulmonary valves and umbilical veins. Heterologous tissues include pericardium, aortic valves and dura mater.

Several metals are also widely used. The sternotomy is almost universally closed with stainless-steel wire. (A number of materials have been used for this purpose over the years, among them linen (long obsolete) and stout monofilament nylon. The nylon is sometimes preferred for babies but the others did not prove to be as satisfactory in the long term as the wire). Many prosthetic heart valves contain some metal, most commonly vitallium, which is an alloy of cobalt and used to make the skeleton of the valve. In one model (see below) the poppet was made of it.

Other, non-metallic substances widely used in heart valves are silicone rubber and pyrolytic carbon. 'Plastic' rings are also used for both mitral and tricuspid annuloplasty.

Heart valves

There is an extremely wide range of prosthetic heart valves available and the list grows longer almost daily; no attempt is made to name them all. Replacement heart valves are classified as either mechanical prostheses or as biological prostheses (often called bioprostheses).

Mechanical prostheses

The earliest mechanical prosthesis was developed in the USA in the 1940s by Hufnagel[1]. It antedated cardiopulmonary bypass, so the operation was done through a lateral thoracotomy; the valve was placed in the descending aorta. A few are still in situ and functioning well[2].

The Bahnson leaflet replacement[3] was introduced for placement in the subcoronary position in 1960. The leaflet was made of a polypropylene material and fashioned to improve the competence of the aortic valve. The modelling of the replacement leaflet was done at the table, during the operation.

The prosthesis of McGoon was a sleeve of knitted Terylene which, like the Bahnson cusp, was fashioned at the table[4].

Caged ball prostheses

In 1960, Starr and his engineer colleague Edwards, both American, introduced the valve which bears their name[5]. The original model had a silicone rubber poppet in a metal cage, with three struts for aortic prostheses and four struts for mitral ones. The sewing ring was (and still is) of silicone foam-rubber covered in knitted cloth. The original model (the 1240) was soon withdrawn because the composition of the poppet permitted the absorption of lipids into it, causing 'ball variance'[6]. The adjustment of the silicone rubber during manufacture abolished ball variance permanently[7] and the modified valve (model 1260) is in worldwide use today.

Efforts to reduce the incidence of thromboembolism in patients with Starr–Edwards valves produced numerous modifications to the basic design. Among these have been: a hollow metal poppet in the original cage; covering the outside of the cage with cloth; covering the seat of the poppet as well as the cage; and covering the seat only. Because the metal poppet has to be placed in the cage before the cage is completed, it is not fully closed at its apex, but the gap is very small.

Other caged ball valves include the Braunwald–Cutter, the Macgovern (which was 'sutureless', being applied with a special instrument which released metal teeth from the valve into the aortic annulus) and the Smeloff–Cutter. They are all slightly different in appearance; for example, in the Braunwald–Cutter the apex of the cage is open with rounded struts.

Tilting disc prostheses

The first tilting disc valve was developed by the Swedish surgeon, Bjork, and the American engineer, Shiley, in 1969[8]. The slightly biconvex disc was 'plastic', while the struts within which the disc tilted were of metal, as was the annulus. The sewing ring, as in all replacement heart valves, was covered in cloth. Like the Starr–Edwards, the Bjork–Shiley valve has undergone modifications, both to improve its haemodynamic characteristics and to reduce the incidence of thromboembolism. The current model is made entirely of pyrolytic carbon and is black.

There have been several other low profile, tilting disc valves but none has been as universally used as the Bjork–Shiley. A few, such as the Hall–Kaster (Norwegian–American) introduced in 1979[9] are in use, but most such as the Hammersmith valve (1964)[10] have long since become obsolete.

Split disc valves

These are also tilting discs but the poppet is split into two equal halves so that when the valve is open the two flaps are at right-angles to the ring, giving a very large orifice, minimally obstructed by the poppet. The poppets are made of pyrolytic carbon. These are relatively new valves so they do not as yet have the multiplicity of model numbers reflecting modifications to the design which all the older ones have. Names include Duromedic, St Jude and Omniscience[11,12].

Bioprostheses

The simplest of the bioprostheses is the 'free' or 'unstented' aortic valve homograft, the use of which was introduced by the New Zealand surgeon Barratt-Boyes in

1962[13]. The valves were collected during necropsy and, in the early days, they were sterilized in β-propriolactone or ethylene oxide gas before storage, either in a tissue culture medium[14–15] or after freeze-drying[16]. Today they are treated by immersion in an antibiotic solution for some days before either freezing or wet storage. Nowadays most aortic valve allografts come from transplantation programmes, and are often used fresh, without any *in vitro* treatment.

Stented homograft valves are sewn into a frame (stent) before further processing.

Heterograft valves are similarly treated; their usual source is the pig, as the size range accords with that of man. These valves are marketed by various manufacturers; some carry the name of a surgeon (for example Carpentier–Edwards), whose ideas were incorporated into the product. The morphology of the stent varies a little according to whether the valve is to be used in the aortic or mitral position, those for the former having a more steeply angled sewing ring. (This also applies to mechanical prostheses.)

In addition to the natural valves, there are several prostheses fashioned from heterologous tissues. They are cut and shaped to resemble the leaflets of aortic valves and are then mounted into a stent. The Wessex Medical valve, for example, was constructed from bovine pericardium. The theory behind these is that they have the advantage of natural valves (lower thrombogenicity) without the restraints imposed by the size of natural ones. However, they are not made in sizes much above 40 mm overall diameter (the orifice is smaller), as the semilunar design, when man made, does not suit larger sizes.

A discussion of the relative merits and deficiencies of mechanical and bioprostheses is beyond the scope of this book but, in the most general terms, mechanical prostheses are durable but more prone to thromboembolic complications than tissue valves. The latter have a limited span *in situ* (about 10 to 15 years) but deteriorate slowly, unlike mechanical valves, which, when they do fail, tend to do so suddenly, with results which may be fatal.

An excellent flow chart to identify some of the prostheses has been devised by Silver and Wilson[17].

Complications: tissue valves versus mechanical valves

Tissue valves are not free from complications but the patient is spared the disadvantages of long-term anticoagulant therapy. Irrespective of their source, tissue valves have a finite life-span, so that all but the oldest patients will eventually need another operation, with all the complications associated with reoperation. The persistence of tissue valves is extremely variable but only rarely exceeds 20 years. The site of implantation is not relevant to persistence *per se*.

Bioprostheses are contraindicated in children and adolescents because the valves were found to calcify early, sometimes within a year. This is usually attributed to a combination of enhanced calcium metabolism and rapid heart rate in young patients.

Endocarditis, both early and late, occurs in bioprostheses, irrespective of their method of preparation and storage. The prevalence rate accords with that for mechanical prostheses.

Bioprostheses are sometimes sent to the laboratory as surgical specimens with a cryptic diagnosis of 'valve failure'. When this occurs early, it is due either to 'valve–patient mismatch' (i.e. it does not fit), to early infective endocarditis or to iatrogenic injury to the valve during insertion. The term 'valve failure' best describes a late complication of tissue valve replacement and is due to degeneration of the prosthesis. This nearly always occurs as a result of thinning of the valve leaflet close to the 'hinge'. In stented valves, the thinning is more noticeable near the commissures, where there is the greatest anatomical distortion of the leaflets (demonstrable with a pulse duplicator), due to hydrodynamic forces acting upon the valve as a whole. Thinning is often accompanied by calcification, usually macroscopic, of the leaflet. Rarely the leaflet (of an aortic valve replacement) may be holed by spicules of calcium from the adjacent mitral valve.

In the case of biograft valves in aortic position, most living patients have a diastolic murmur by the end of the first year following operation, so that a degree of regurgitation is nearly always present. This regurgitation causes turbulence, which in turn causes a degree of haemolysis. Obviously, severe haemolytic anaemia necessitates a change of valve, but the hepatic, splenic and renal manifestations of subclinical haemolysis are often to be seen at necropsy. In unstented grafts there is no possibility for paravalvular leaks, as there is no paravalvular space, so that in the absence of infection deterioration of the graft must be suspected as a cause of regurgitation. Valve failure is a slow and (usually) gradual process, so that a relatively grossly abnormal valve may be found at necropsy, especially in old people. However, sudden spontaneous leaflet rupture is a rare cause of late death in patients with tissue valves.

Tissue valves in atrioventricular position are obligatorily stented, adding to the prosthetic material in the heart and theoretically loading the risk of endocarditis. Most valves for this purpose are heterograft (usually porcine) aortic valves, inverted and stented. Hence they are of limited size, so that in all but the smallest patients there is likely to be a degree of mitral stenosis.

Viability of tissue valves

Commercially produced valves are tanned in glutaraldehyde, so that for practical purposes they are immunologically and biologically inert. Glutaraldehyde has a sterilizing action as well as that of stabilizing protein. The mode of stabilization is uncertain, but glutaraldehyde permits more, and more stable, cross-linkages in collagen than do other aldehydes[18]. Eventually these cross-linkages weaken, and the degenerating collagen calcifies.

By contrast, homograft valves are often treated by immersion in solutions of antibiotics, and may still be viable at the time of insertion. There have been sporadic reports of immune reaction to such valves, but as they are quickly replaced in such cases the patients rarely come to necropsy. Homograft valves collected aseptically (e.g. during transplantation procedures) can be implanted without further treatment, and these valves may precipitate rejection. There are anecdotal accounts of such 'fresh' homografts having survived for a number of years, as shown by neutrophil morphology, but this is not generally the case.

Mechanical prostheses

Non-tissue valves have the advantage of greater durability but the patients require lifelong anticoagulant therapy, with its attendant morbidity. Many late deaths are due to complications of anticoagulation, notably cerebral haemorrhage.

Haemolysis is another disadvantage of mechanical valves. This is largely due to turbulence resulting from transvalvular pressure gradients, and is more severe in caged ball valves than in tilting disc models.

References

1. Hufnagel, C. A., Harvey, W. P., Rabil, P. J. and McDermott, T. F. Surgical correction of aortic insufficiency. *Surgery*, **35**, 673–683, 1954
2. Hufnagel, C. A. and Gomes, M. N. Late follow-up of ball valve prostheses in the descending thoracic aorta. *Journal of Thoracic and Cardiovascular Surgery*, **72**, 900–909, 1976
3. Bahnson, H. T., Spencer, F. C., Busse, E. F. G. and Davis, F. W. Jr. Cusp replacement and coronary artery perfusion in open operations on the aortic valve. *Annals of Surgery*, **152**, 494–505, 1960
4. McGoon, D. C. Acquired aortic valve disease. *Surgery*, **53**, 372–386, 1963
5. Starr, A. and Edwards, M. L. Mitral replacement; clinical experience with a ball valve prosthesis. *Annals of Surgery*, **154**, 726–740, 1961
6. Krosnick, A. Death due to migration of the ball from an aortic valve prosthesis. *Journal of the American Medical Association*, **191**, 1083–1084, 1965
7. Hylen, J. C., Kloster, F. E., Starr, A. and Griswold, H. E. Aortic ball variance; diagnosis and treatment. *Annals of Internal Medicine*, **71**, 1–8, 1970
8. Bjork, V. O. A new tilting disc prosthesis. *Scandinavian Journal of Cardiovascular Surgery*, **3**, 1–10, 1969
9. Hall, K. V., Kaster, R. L. and Woien, A. An improved disc type heart valve design. *Journal of the Oslo City Hospitals*, **29**, 3–21, 1979
10. Melrose, D. G., Bentall, H. H., McMillan, I. K. R. *et al.* Evolution of a mitral valve prosthesis. *Lancet*, **ii**, 623–624, 1964
11. Emery, R. W., Palmquist, W. E., Mettler, E. and Nicoloff, D. M. A new cardiac valve prosthesis. *In vitro* results. *Transactions of the American Society for Artificial Internal Organs*, **24**, 550–556, 1978
12. Barratt-Boyes, B. G. Homograft aortic valve replacement in aortic incompetence and stenosis. *Thorax*, **19**, 131–150, 1964
13. Rains, A. J. H., Crawford, N., Sharp, S. H. *et al.* Management of an artery graft bank with special reference to β-propriolactone. *Lancet*, **ii**, 830–832, 1956
14. Gross, R. E., Bill, A. H. and Pierce, E. C. Methods of preserving and transplantation of arterial grafts. Observations of arterial grafts in dogs. Report of transplantation of preserved arterial grafts in 9 human cases. *Surgery, Gynecology and Obstetrics*, **88**, 689–701, 1949
15. Barratt-Boyes, B. G. Long-term follow-up of aortic valvar grafts. *British Heart Journal*, **Supplement 33**, 60–65, 1971
16. Allwork, S. P., Pucci, J. J., Cleland, W. P. and Bentall, H. H. The longevity of sterilised aortic valve homografts 1966–1972. *Journal of Cardiovascular Surgery*, **27**, 213–216, 1986
17. Silver, M. D. and Wilson, G. J. Pathology of cardiovascular prostheses including coronary artery bypass and other vascular grafts. In *Cardiovascular Pathology*, vol. 2 (ed. M. D. Silver), Churchill Livingstone, New York, pp. 1225–1296, 1983
18. Woodruff, E. A. The chemistry and biology of aldehyde treated tissue heart valve xenografts. In *Tissue Valves* (ed. M. J. Ionescu), Butterworths, London, p. 347, 1979

3

Valve operations and post-mortem findings

Valve operations

About one-third of cardiac surgical procedures are accounted for by valve operations.

Mitral valve operations

Closed mitral valvotomy

This is now a rare operation. It is performed without cardiopulmonary bypass (hence 'closed'), as follows: left thoracotomy, left atriotomy through the appendage, apical left ventriculotomy controlled with a purse-string. The valve orifice is measured and a dilator, set to the desired size, is advanced (closed) through the left ventricle to the stenosed valve, into which it is introduced and then opened. This manoeuvre is repeated until the required orifice is achieved. The left atrial appendage is ligated and the ventriculotomy closed. Drains are laid and the chest closed in layers.

Open mitral valvotomy

This has largely superseded the closed procedure, at least in the UK. (The exception is during pregnancy: the closed operation is quick and does not subject the fetus to the risk of ischaemia during bypass.) The open procedure also permits annuloplasty and the refashioning of the valve leaflets as alternatives to valve replacement. Open valvotomy (or annuloplasty) is done under cardiopulmonary bypass, through a median sternotomy. The left atrium is incised directly.

Annuloplasty

In this operation (approached as above) the valve ring is reduced either by placing a purse-string around part of it (Wooler's operation), by placing a double purse-string around the annulus and adjusting the tension to the desired diameter (De Vega's annuloplasty) or by fitting a soft plastic ring and tailoring the valve to that (Carpentier's annuloplasty). The leaflets are also amenable to refashioning.

Leaflet resection

In addition to the above, there is another procedure especially suitable for mitral valve regurgitation due to causes other than rheumatic heart disease (e.g. ruptured chordae tendineae). In this, a section of the valve is excised as a rectangle of tissue comprising the affected chordae, the adjacent leaflet and a small segment of annulus (Figure 3.1). The edges of the remaining annulus and leaflet are apposed and sutured so that competence of the valve is restored.

Mitral valve replacement (median sternotomy, cardiopulmonary bypass)

The mitral valve may be approached either directly through the left atrium or via the atrial septum through a right atriotomy. The latter is sometimes preferred if the tricuspid valve is to be operated upon as well. The anterior leaflet of the valve is excised in its entirety, together with the chordae tendineae and some or all of the

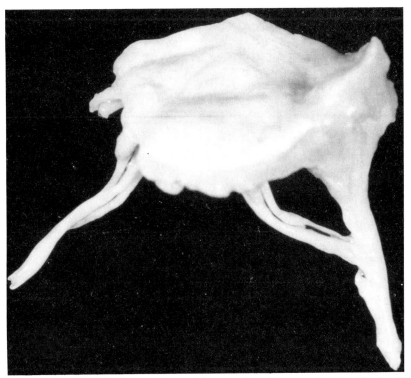

Figure 3.1 Surgical specimen of wedge excision of scallop of the posterior mitral leaflet. Mitral valve regurgitation was due to ruptured chordae tendineae (seen on the left)

anterior papillary muscle group. The posterior leaflet and its tensor apparatus are often left *in situ*. The new valve may be placed with either interrupted or continuous sutures, the interrupted technique is as follows: a double-ended suture is placed through the annulus and through the prosthesis in such a manner that there are two 'bites' through both; the ends are tied with several knots as the suture material is slippery and the knots may unravel unless they are well secured. This technique applies equally to all valve replacements. Continuous sutures are placed at the edge of the prosthesis with the second 'bite' more towards the centre. The atriotomy (and septum, which is sometimes incised to approach the left atrium (Dubost's incision), if used) is closed with a continuous suture.

Aortic valve operations

The aortic valve is approached (on bypass), through a J-shaped or hockey-stick incision extending from just above the right aortic sinus to a convenient place in the ascending aorta.

Aortic valvotomy is almost entirely confined to the paediatric patents with congenital malformations, but it is sometimes feasible in adult patients. The fused commissures are incised under direct vision.

Débridement of calcium is sometimes feasible. Calcium is removed from the valve with both blunt and sharp dissection, with a pack placed in the left ventricle to catch any particles of calcium. At the end, the aorta is closed with continuous suture.

Konno's operation for aortic valve regurgitation[1]: the leaflets of the aortic valve are resuspended by placing a stay stitch through the noduli Arantii, then resecting and stitching until the leaflets coapt in diastole.

Aortic valve replacement: the native valve is removed close to its annulus; if there is annular calcification, as much as is practicable is removed, together with any 'candle wax' runs of calcium on to the anterior leaflet of the mitral valve. If the aortic root is small it may be increased in diameter by incising the area of aortomitral continuity and inserting a wedge-shaped gusset of material, which may be either pericardium or cloth. An alternative technique is to incise the infundibular septum, sacrificing one or two of the pulmonary valve leaflets and inserting a gusset, as above. (Also described by Konno[2].)

Although these two procedures are perhaps more often associated with the treatment of congenitally small aortic root (e.g. in Turner's syndrome), both have a place in the management of acquired aortic valve stenosis as well.

The new aortic valve is placed with interrupted sutures. In the case of unstented homografts, there are two suture lines: the first below the leaflets, and the second securing the pillars of graft aorta and aortic sinuses. The aortotomy is closed, often over pledgets of felt, with a continuous suture.

Replacement of the aortic valve and ascending aorta

Wheat's operation[3]: the valve is replaced, then the ascending aorta is excised leaving the coronary arteries in place. The ascending aorta is then replaced with a graft. The native aorta is usually retained to wrap the graft.

'Classical' Bentall's operation[4]: a composite graft is prepared by sewing a prosthesis into a cloth graft. This is then implanted and at the same time the coronary arteries are reimplanted through the graft. The native aorta is used to wrap the graft.

'Modified' Bentall's operation: if the aortic root is so large that reimplantation is impractical, vein grafts are used to bridge the gap. The native aorta is wrapped around the graft and, in addition, a stoma may be made in the aorta, which is then anastomosed to the right atrium to afford a drain. Both mechanical and biological valves are suitable for this operation.

Because operations to replace the aortic root are so particularly associated with the treatment of infective endocarditis, they are described in Chapter 4.

Multiple valve operations

As the incidence of new rheumatic heart disease continues to decline, the necessity for multiple valve replacements declines with it. Although triple valve replacement is now a fairly rare procedure (41 of 5026 valve operations in 1984), aortic and mitral replacements still accounted for 613 operations in the same year, while mitral and tricuspid replacements numbered 120. A combination of, say, aortic replacement and a conservative mitral procedure offers an alternative. The combination of aortic and tricuspid replacement is uncommon (seven in 1984)[5].

Tricuspid valve operations

Organic tricuspid valve disease is uncommon even as part of the spectrum of rheumatic heart disease, and is rare on its own. Replacement of the valve may be necessary in the treatment of end-stage rheumatic disease but, as already indicated, the need is decreasing steadily. Annuloplasty is performed whenever possible. When replacement is unavoidable, bioprostheses tend to be preferred to mechanical valves for the tricuspid position. This is partly due to the shape of the tricuspid annulus and right ventricle, and partly because the thrombogenicity of mechanical valves is increased in the tricuspid position[6].

Tricuspid valve replacement may still be performed for infective endocarditis or for a congenital malformation. In the case of endocarditis, the tricuspid valve is commonly affected in abusers of drugs, especially those taking them intravenously; it is also at risk in patients with long-term intravenous lines and those with transvenous endocardial pacemakers (see also Chapter 4).

The operation is done (on bypass) through a right atriotomy. Either suture technique may be used.

Post-mortem assessment of valve replacement

Mitral valve operations

Closed mitral valvotomy

In closed mitral valvotomy there are two chief causes of *early death*: firstly, tamponade due to iatrogenic cardiac rupture and, secondly, acute pulmonary oedema due to mitral regurgitation caused either by accidental detachment of a leaflet from the annulus or by overdilatation. These complications were more or less confined to patients with valves unsuitable for closed mitral valvotomy in the days before preoperative assessment was as good as it is today. Now, with excellent diagnostic facilities, e.g. two-dimensional echocardiography, it is unlikely that a patient with a calcified valve (the usual cause of the catastrophies outlined above) would have been offered this operation, and modern interoperative pressure monitoring would normally prevent excessive dilatation.

Late death is likely to be due to mitral restenosis and the effects of progress of the disease. The anticipated findings are as follows:

1. Lateral thoractomy.
2. Absent left atrial appendage.
3. Small apical ventriculotomy scar.
4. Left atrial enlargement, indicative of mitral regurgitation.
5. No left atrial enlargement, indicative of stenosis only.
6. Calcified mitral annulus, especially in older patients.
7. Loss of characteristic mitral valve morphology.
8. Thickening, and sometimes calcification, of the leaflets.
9. Fusion and shrinkage of the chordae tendineae.
10. Macroscopic fibrosis of the papillary muscles.
11. 'Rheumatic' changes in the aortic valve.
12. 'Rheumatic' changes in the tricuspid valve.
13. Biventricular hypertrophy and diffuse myocardial fibrosis.
14. Dilatation of the pulmonary valve and pulmonary artery.
15. (Coronary artery disease.)

Open mitral valvotomy

This is a low-risk operation so that deaths *early* in the postoperative period are rare. If they do occur, the cause is most likely to be due to complications of cardiopulmonary bypass (see Chapter 1). Haemorrhage is the most likely of these complications, as some patients, anticoagulated because of atrial fibrillation, develop a bleeding diathesis when subjected to cardiopulmonary bypass, which does respond to the medications usually successful in non-surgical patients.

In *late deaths*, the anticipated findings are: a midline scar plus the abnormalities listed in (3)–(14) above. As in all older patients, coronary artery disease may also be implicated, and may supersede the ongoing effects of rheumatic heart disease.

It is usually impossible to identify a plane of cleavage, or to determine what had been done to the valve at operation, when death occurs late (months or years) after operation.

Annuloplasty

Like open valvotomy, this is a low-risk operation so that deaths *early* in the postoperative period are likely to be attributable to a complication of bypass. *Late death*, particularly if the operation was not for rheumatic heart disease, may be due to an unrelated cause.

In the De Vega type of annuloplasty the repair is sometimes visible as lengths of suture in the annulus but more often there is nothing of the operation to be seen, unless the annulus is dissected meticulously, as the thread is deep in the sulcus tissue. The suture line apposing the cut edges of the leaflet in the wedge excision type of repair can be identified in non-rheumatic hearts by slight thickening of the leaflet and sometimes by the cut ends of the sutures on the atrial aspect of the leaflet. If the whole valve is thickened the operation site may be identifiable only by careful palpation. Other findings are as described for mitral valvotomy.

Mitral valve replacement

Repeat cardiac surgery has a high operative mortality and mitral valve replacement is sometimes a third, fourth or even fifth operation.

Early death

Early death after mitral valve replacement can be due to any of the complications of bypass, particularly haemorrhage. In addition to these there are some events peculiar to the operation.

Rupture of the left ventricle   When this occurs within the first 24 h after operation there are two likely sites: the first is the mitral annulus itself; the most vulnerable place is the posterior segment, particularly if the patient had had previous operations on the mitral valve. The surgical approach to these necessitates some manipulation of the back of the heart, which sometimes heals with dense adhesions both in the pericardium and in the lung. (This is especially well exemplified by patients with a history of multiple mitral valvotomies and old pulmonary tuberculosis.) At replacement, attempts to divide adhesions can cause lacerations of the left ventricle (which is of only normal thickness in 'pure' mitral stenosis), which then continue to tear, causing eventual rupture. It is to reduce this risk that the posterior mitral leaflet and its tensor apparatus are often not excised during the operation.

The second site of left ventricular rupture is the stump of the papillary muscles, particularly the posterior group. Again, patients with stenosis only are most at risk. If tension is put on the chordae tendineae during surgical excision of the valve, when the heart is arrested and relaxed by cardioplegia, there is a risk of cutting a little 'buttonhole' in the wall of the left ventricle. This laceration then proceeds to a larger one which is almost impossible to rescue once heartbeat is restored.

Of course both these hazards are very well recognized by surgeons, and fatal left ventricular rupture from either of them is a relatively rare cause of perioperative death.

When left ventricular rupture occurs at 7–10 days after operation the cause is likely to be myocardial necrosis. The most common precedent for this is preoperative or interoperative myocardial infarction. Many patients have concomitant coronary artery disease and sometimes operation is expedited by a sudden deterioration in their condition which is attributed to the valve disease. The effects of perfusion and cardiac manipulation make interoperative myocardial infarction notoriously difficult to diagnose biochemically and electrocardiographic-ally, so that the histopathologist has an almost unparalleled opportunity to make as perfect as possible a temporal clinicopathological correlation.

A less common cause of myocardial necrosis relates directly to the valve replacement. If there is heavy calcification the valve may be difficult to excise. Either the calcium itself or the dissection to excise the valve can lacerate the endocardium of the left ventricle; the area subjacent to the aortomitral continuity is the most vulnerable. The laceration exposes the subendocardium, itself a region liable to ischaemic damage, and necrosis spreads in a spiral course towards the apex. Up to about 40% of the left ventricle can become necrotic by this means, even when there is no coronary artery disease.

Accidental coronary artery occlusion   Although both the length and the diameter of the circumflex branch of the left coronary artery are extremely variable[7], its location in the left atrioventricular sulcus is constant. This sulcus is covered by the epicardium and a variable amount of fat. The great cardiac vein traverses it, usually but not always superficial to the circumflex branch, which lies deep in the sulcus, close to the annulus fibrosus of the mitral valve. Haematoma in the sulcus indicates that the great cardiac vein was pierced during the operation and is a frequent finding after mitral valve replacement. Hence it is hardly surprising that very occasionally the circumflex branch is accidentally caught in a stitch being placed to anchor the new valve. This mishap may be of little or no consequence if the circumflex branch is short and small, but may cause massive infarction in an individual with a dominant left coronary artery. The circumflex branch in these people is often larger than the anterior descending branch[7]. The cause of the accident is invisible to the surgeon, so that if it is suspected at the end of the operation, the valve must be taken out and replaced anew, by which time myocardial infarction may already have occurred.

Myocardial contusion   Laceration and haemorrhage in the septum is sometimes observed at the site of the impact with the valve struts but is of no clinical consequence. It is particularly noticeable in patients with normal-sized ventricles, but it seems to be of little or no significance in that it does not interfere with conduction. The site heals as a patch of thickened endocardium.

Late death
Mechanical valves seldom 'fail' in the sense of falling apart of breaking, but some models can wear: for example, the cloth over the struts of some Starr–Edwards valves can become partly detached (a common finding after several years). The hazards late after replacement are infective endocarditis and thromboembolism.

Infective endocarditis   The relatively new disease of prosthetic valve endocarditis is considered in more detail in Chapter 4. All patients with prosthetic valves are at risk from it and the infection can affect the natural valves as well. Endocarditis affects the patient's anticoagulant control when the illness is terminal so that there may be ante-mortem thrombus partially or totally occluding the valve.

Thromboembolism   All patients with artificial heart valves are at risk from thromboembolism. The risk of thrombosis may be reduced when improved design and materials for prosthetic valves become available. At necropsy there may be little on the valve itself to point to the cause, and the prosthesis may look quite normal (that is, it is well healed, without thrombi adhering to it, it moves through its full excursion and there are neither loose suture ends nor paraprosthetic leaks).

The ideal way to examine the heart is to follow the procedure given in Chapter 1 but, before fixing the heart, open the left atrium and rinse away obvious post-mortem thrombus so that the valve is well displayed. Usually the cut suture ends are still faintly visible through the neointima. If there are patches without neointima a paraprosthetic leak should be suspected, with sepsis as its cause. Note the position of the valve poppet and whether it moves freely or is obstructed by thrombus or vegetation. If there is a significant paraprosthetic leak it is usually easy to see from the atrium. Gentle probing at this stage will indicate the extent of the gap. If there is no obvious hole but one had been suspected or identified in life it is likely to originate in the ventricle. Despite wishing to find it as quickly as possible, it will be more easily and accurately located if the search is postponed until the specimen has been fixed.

Having opened the ventricle to display both inflow and outflow portions, any cavities around the mitral annulus should be plainly visible. Small holes may tunnel into the myocardium, forming the cavity which was diagnosed in life. Chronic paraprosthetic leaks are usually easy to identify from the left atrium, and the degree of healing of the prosthesis can be assessed (Figures 3.2 and 3.3). Caged ball valves produce patches of endocardial thickening where the struts of the cage impinge upon the septum and free wall of the left ventricle, and in the (now obsolete) models with cloth-covered struts a thick pseudointima often accompanies cloth wear (Figure 3.4).

If there are no major findings such as those above, the anticipated appearances of the heart late after mechanical prosthetic mitral valve replacement are:

1. Cardiomegaly (almost invariably).
2. Endocardial thickening in the left ventricular outflow tract, especially where there is a caged ball prosthesis.
3. Incorporation of the struts of the cage into the free wall.
4. Wear of the cloth in a cloth-covered cage.

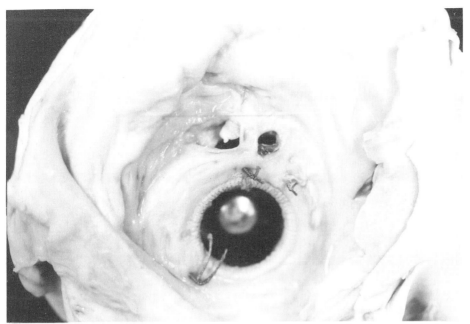

Figure 3.2 Starr–Edwards metal ball valve in mitral position. There are two chronic paraprosthetic leaks; some long suture ends are still visible after 10 years. The seat of the valve is poorly healed, and the iatrogenic mitral stenosis is reflected in the relative dilatation of the left atrium and the endocardial thickening of the chamber

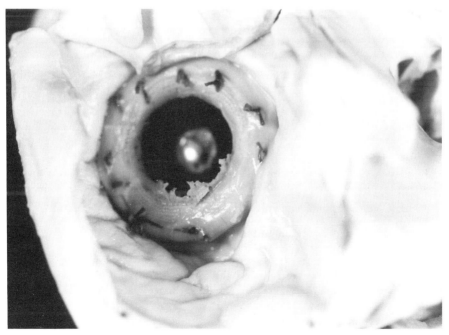

Figure 3.3 Poorly healed metal ball valve in mitral position. There is a paraprosthetic leak at 6 o'clock, and pannus extending from 3 to 7 o'clock

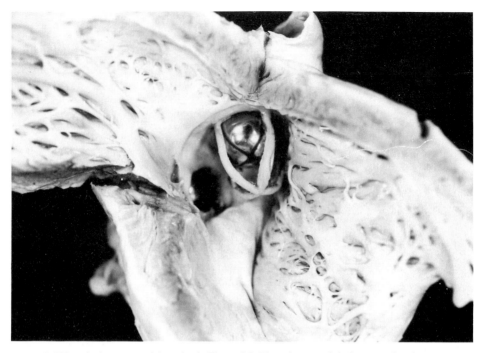

Figure 3.4 Ventricular aspect of the valve in Figure 3.3. There is a pseudointima covering the struts, together with some cloth wear. There are patches of endocardial thickening both on the septum and on the posterior wall of the left ventricle. The posterior leaflet of the native mitral valve was not excised during operation

5. Findings consistent with long-standing rheumatic heart disease in the other valves.
6. Coronary artery disease.

Replacement with tissue valves
In early death, the comments on mechanical valve replacement apply equally to tissue valves as do those concerning the examination of the heart.

All tissue valves, irrespective of material, are small by comparison with the atrioventricular orifice into which they are placed. The size (e.g. 35 mm) refers to the overall diameter *not* the orifice, which is considerably smaller. Therefore, all patients with this type of valve have a greater or lesser degree of mitral stenosis, and often the pathology (e.g. pulmonary hypertension) associated with it, when they come to post-mortem late after operation.

Tissue valves wear out after 10–15 years in mature adults, so that thinning of the leaflets, sometimes into holes, is to be anticipated. They also calcify. Bioprostheses are contraindicated in children and young people because of early calcification, sometimes necessitating another replacement within a year[8].

These valves are less thrombogenic than mechanical valves but thromboembolism may occur, and the valve itself may be thrombosed, particularly in the presence of infection.

Aortic valve operations

Whereas most mitral valve operations are for rheumatic heart disease, many aortic valve replacements are for other reasons. Infective endocarditis is considered in Chapter 4 but other predisposing conditions are congenital aortic valve stenosis and aortic valve stenosis due to calcification in mature life.

Early death after operation is likely to be the result of complications of bypass. Haemorrhage is a particular hazard, as the patients are often among the oldest surgical patients and may be in the eighth or ninth decade of life. The combination of poststenotic dilatation and loss of elastic in the aorta predisposes to postoperative bleeding from the aortotomy.

The other major cause of early death, especially in the elderly, is myocardial infarction. (However, operations to revascularize do not significantly increase the operative risk; see Chapter 5.) Calcific coronary embolization is not a great hazard as the coronary arteries are usually cannulated for coronary perfusion or cardioplegia, so that fragments of calcium cannot escape into that system. Dissection of a coronary artery after cannulation is rare in patients without genetic connective tissue disorders.

A rare cause of early death is accidental occlusion of an aberrant coronary artery. Positional anomalies of the coronary ostia occur fairly frequently in congenitally bicuspid aortic valve, and are found in about 2% of otherwise congenitally normal hearts[9]. An ostium placed low in the aortic sinus may escape search (for cannulation) at operation, particularly if there is heavy calcification, and being undetected is then liable to be occluded by the sewing ring of the valve.

The other anomaly which may be implicated in early postoperative death is origin of a coronary artery from an inappropriate aortic sinus. The aberrant artery is likely to pass between the aorta and the pulmonary artery and be occluded if there is a sharp rise in blood pressure, as sometimes happens in the first hours after operation. Massive infarction results. It may seem strange that such anomalies are not invariably identified before operation; policy about coronary arteriography in aortic valve disease varies very considerably among cardiological centres and, in addition, the aberrations may be masked by massive calcification.

The degree of diffuse fibrosis of the left ventricle may be striking, even in the absence of coronary artery disease, particularly in patients whose aortic valves were both stenotic and regurgitant.

In *late death* an often impressive finding is the weight of the heart, particularly if the replacement had been for regurgitation rather than stenosis.

Even in late death the aortotomy may be implicated: a slow leak can cause tamponade 6 months or more after operation. Such leaks may appear as false aneurysms. They are not necessarily associated with sepsis, but it is often implicated.

When there is gross hypertrophy, the valve is sometimes difficult to examine, even from the left ventricle; it is often almost impossible from above (i.e. the aorta) unless there is marked dilatation of the aorta. To overcome this, open the aorta down to the valve ring, noting the position of the coronary ostia. The cage of a Starr–Edwards valve should appear bright and without neointima; the cloth-covered models (no longer being implanted) may have shreds of the cloth hanging from the cage if they have been there a long time. Both metal (in the cloth-covered model) and silicone rubber poppets (the model 1260, most often used) are also bright and perfectly spherical; the suture ends may still be visible through the neointima covering the sewing ring.

Paraprosthetic leaks are not usually easy to see from the aorta, so gentle probing around the annulus is appropriate. If there is a leak, its position may be indicated by a Zahn–Schminker pocket in the outflow tract of the left ventricle. Paraprosthetic leaks point to infective endocarditis but where infected allograft valves are concerned such leaks do not occur because the absence of a stent means that there is no paravalvular space. If there is a leak, its presence may be indicated by a small lesion, facing the valve, in the endocardium of the left ventricular outflow tract. This is a focus of endocardial fibrosis which develops at the site where a jet of abnormally directed blood impinges on the myocardium. Sometimes these jet lesions resemble a watch pocket, facing the stream. Jet lesions with this morphology are called Zahn–Schminker pockets and pinpoint the location of the leak (Figure 3.5).

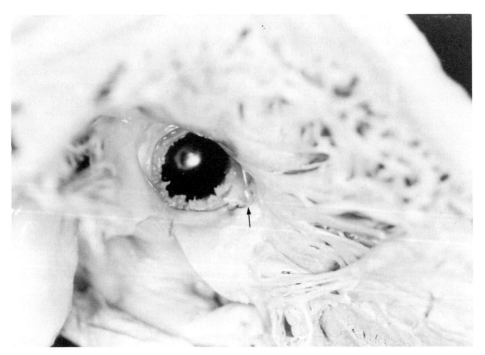

Figure 3.5 In addition to pannus, there is a jet lesion (arrowed) tunnelling into the area of aortomitral continuity

When examined from the ventricle the valve ring is clothed with neointima. If this neointima extends a little over the ring, to obstruct the orifice to a small degree, either sepsis or thrombus formation should be suspected, but a modest endocardial thickening (up to about 1 mm) of the outflow tract immediately subjacent to the valve is normal for these patients (Figure 3.6). If the valve is thrombosed it is easy to see. If the thrombus is accompanied by major dehiscence the whole prosthesis rocks in the outflow tract (Figure 3.7).

In late deaths with 'successful' valve replacements, when death is due to other causes, the anticipated findings are as follows:

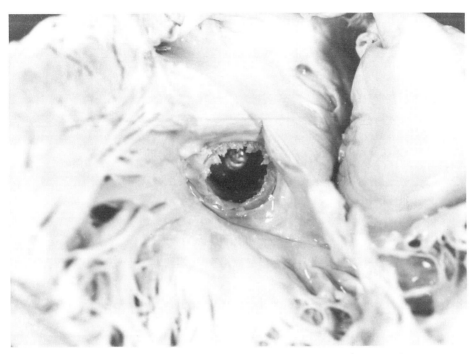

Figure 3.6 Left ventricular view of aortic valve prosthesis. The valve is infected and there is a paraprosthetic leak, as well as pannus and slight thickening subjacent to the leak. (The anterior mitral leaflet has been divided)

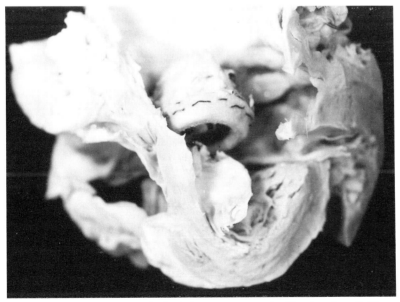

Figure 3.7 Aortic prosthesis attached only by two sutures to the dilated aortic wall. The prosthesis, in an involucrum of thrombus, was rocking in the aorta, the whole acting as a valve

1. Midline chest wound.
2. Aortotomy sometimes visible.
3. Prosthetic valve bright, no leaks, no thrombus, moving freely.
4. No Zahn–Schminker pockets in the left ventricular outflow tract.
5. No vegetations.
6. Cardiomegaly.
7. Left ventricular hypertrophy.
8. (Coronary artery disease.)
9. (Calcium extending across the ventricular aspect of the anterior leaflet of the mitral valve.)
10. (Calcification of the mitral annulus.)

Left ventricular hypertrophy is almost universal in these patients. Where there was dilatation before operation, the heart may be heavier than in patients with stenosis alone. Neither weighing the heart nor measuring wall thickness gives a really accurate indication of ventricular hypertrophy. Weight is related to mass, but wall thickness depends on the volume of the chambers and the muscle bulk. These variables may be affected by a number of factors, such as fixation techniques and whether the heart stopped in systole or diastole.

If accurate assessment is necessary, the method whereby the ventricles are separated and weighed separately, with the septum being assigned to the left ventricle (Fulton's method), should be used. The septum increases in weight with the left ventricle, and not if the right is hypertrophied. The technique has the obvious drawback of destroying the morphology of the specimen.

Microscopic assessment of hypertrophy can be done by measuring the diameter of the myocardial fibres. There is no mitosis in myocardial cells in adults, and man has the full complement of cells at an early age, so that, theoretically at least, increasing mass is due to increasing cell size. However, an important factor affecting fibre diameter is increasing cavity volume, which stretches the fibres, giving the appearance of narrowing.

Replacement of the aortic valve and ascending aorta

Early deaths, as in all other cardiac operations, are likely to be associated with the complications of bypass. For all that there is such an apparent potential for bleeding through the graft, early tamponade is uncommon. The grafts are usually 'pre-clotted' and the native aorta is wrapped around the graft so that the potential for catastrophic haemorrhage is thereby much reduced. More often, early death is related to the pre-existing poor haemodynamic status of the patient: these operations are often emergency procedures for dissection or even rupture.

Aneurysms of the ascending aorta are associated with genetic disorders of collagen and elastic tissue, as well as with bicuspid aortic valve, coarctation of the aorta and some tropical infections (notably yaws). There are thus numerous entities predisposing to early death, in addition to those complicating cardiopulmonary bypass.

Patients with Marfan's disease are prone to arrhythmias and are frequently maintained on β-blockers, which can be inimical to 'weaning-off' cardiopulmonary bypass. It is difficult to identify a cause for death at necropsy in these patients.

Peroperative or perioperative myocardial infarction is rare in younger patients, such as those with Marfan's disease or other genetic anomalies, but they are not exempt from intraluminal coronary artery disease. Intimal hyperplasia of both the large epicardial branches and the intramuscular arteries is a striking feature in Marfan's disease, even at a young age (teens and twenties). Furthermore, these patients often have small coronary arteries; in normal adult men the anterior descending branch of the left coronary artery is seldom less than 4 mm in diameter in its proximal portion, whereas in Marfan's disease the author has often observed that the vessel measures no more than 2–3 mm.

Although *late death* may be due to the other manifestations of Marfan's disease, those concerning the heart are the most likely to be implicated. The aorta feels firm and stiff, due to the overwrapping of the graft. The suture line may be visible. If the coronary arteries were reimplanted without vein grafts they are not prominent, but if grafts were used these may appear as rather large vessels and are thus conspicuous, especially in Marfan's disease. In this condition late death may often be attributable to dissection, either of the aorta or of a coronary artery (usually the left). False aneurysms can occur at either end of the graft; these may permit communication between the aortic root and the graft so that there is a continuous leakage of blood into the space between the graft and the wrap of native aorta. True aneurysms may develop in other parts of the aorta or in any other artery and may rupture or dissect, or both, as do those of other aetiologies.

In order to examine the valve replacement it is usually necessary to incise both graft and native aorta down to the sewing ring, taking care not to damage the reimplanted or grafted coronary arteries. The prosthetic valve should be bright, moving fully and be unobstructed by pannus or thrombus. The mitral valve is susceptible to myxomatous degeneration, even in young people, and may be much dilated. The tricuspid valve may also be affected, but less severely so. Myocardial fibrosis and foci of very recent myocardial necrosis are often found in the absence of discrete infarction, which is relatively uncommon in these patients, who are often young.

In patients with other arterial diseases, intraluminal coronary artery disease and recent myocardial infarction are anticipated findings, while aneurysms are less common.

References

1. Konno, S., Yasubaru, I., Yoshimao, I. *et al.* A new method for prosthetic valve replacement in congenital aortic stenosis associated with hypoplasia of the aortic valve. *Journal of Thoracic and Cardiovascular Surgery,* **70**, 909–917, 1975
2. Harlam, B. J., Starr, A. and Harrison, F. M. In *Manual of Cardiac Surgery*, vol. 2, Springer Verlag, New York, p. 223, 1981
3. Wheat, M. E. Jr. Treatment of dissecting aneurysms of the aorta. *Annals of Thoracic Surgery,* **12**, 582–592, 1971
4. Bentall, H. H. and DeBono, A. A technique for complete replacement of the ascending aorta. *Thorax,* **23**, 338–339, 1968
5. Society of Thoracic and Cardiovascular Surgeons of Great Britain and Ireland. *Returns of the UK Cardiac Surgery Register,* 1984
6. Grondin, P., Meere, C., Linet, C. *et al.* Carpentier's annulus and DeVega's annuloplasty. The end of the tricuspid challenge. *Journal of Thoracic and Cardiovascular Surgery,* **70**, 852–861, 1975
7. Allwork, S. P. The anatomy of the coronary arteries. In *The Surgery of Coronary Artery Disease* (ed. D. J. Wheatley), Chapman and Hall, London, pp. 15–25, 1986
8. Silver, M. M., Pollock, J. and Silver, M. D. Calcification of porcine xenografts in children. *American Journal of Cardiology,* **45**, 685–689, 1980
9. Ogden, J. Congenital anomalies of the coronary arteries. *American Journal of Cardiology,* **25**, 474–479, 1970

4

Infective endocarditis

Infective endocarditis is generally a 'medical' rather than a 'surgical' disease but, in the author's Institution, it accounts for approximately 1.8% of valve operations[1]. The conditions, both cardiovascular and others, which predispose to infective endocarditis are listed in Table 4.1. The term 'infective' is preferred to 'bacterial', as organisms other than bacteria (for example, *Rickettsia*, *Chlamydia*) may be responsible for the infection. Furthermore, mixed infections occur, particularly in prosthetic valve endocarditis (PVE).

Table 4.1 Factors which do/do not predispose to infective endocarditis

Cardiovascular factors predisposing to infective endocarditis
Regurgitant valves
  Rheumatic
    Myxomatous
  Degenerative
   'Floppy'
  Marfan's disease
  Hypertrophic obstructive cardiomyopathy
Bicuspid aortic valves
Discrete subaortic stenosis
Small ventricular septal defect
Patent ductus arteriosus
Coarctation of the aorta
Arteriovenous fistula
Prosthetic heart valves
Intracardiac foreign bodies

Cardiovascular factors not predisposing to infective endocarditis
Stenotic valves
Atrial septal defect
Large ventricular septal defect
Prosthetic arterial grafts
Aortocoronary vein bypass grafts

Non-cardiovascular factors predisposing to infective endocarditis
Alcoholism
Old age
Uraemia
Chronic haemodialysis
Immunosuppressive therapy
Intravenous drug addiction

At necropsy, the task is to locate the infection and to identify vegetations, abscesses, abscess cavities and mycotic and ruptured aneurysms, as well as areas of septic necrosis and septic emboli. The sites and types of lesions are given in Table 4.2. Although there are spectacular means of intracardiac imaging to facilitate diagnosis, they are for the most part disappointingly unhelpful in this disease. Vegetations, the *sine qua non* of infected valves, can develop at an extremely rapid rate. In addition they are friable and may embolize, and in PVE they are not usually detectable by two-dimensional (2D)-echocardiography. Similarly, the extent of cavities is often unclear, both by this means and by angiocardiography. Simple fluoroscopy readily identifies a rocking prosthesis but cannot demonstrate the tissue damage which the rocking may have caused. Discrete cavities and

Table 4.2 Location and types of lesion in infective endocarditis

Location		Lesions
Aortic Mitral } valve leaflets		Vegetations, holes, tears, aneurysms
Aortic Mitral } annuli		Abscesses, aneurysms, rupture
Myocardium		Abscesses, aneurysms, rupture, microinfarcts, inflammatory lesions
Tricuspid Pulmonary } valves		Vegetations, holes, tears
Pericardium		Abscesses, rupture

paravalvular leaks, especially small ones, tend to remain unrecognized. The abscesses themselves, and their extent, are often very difficult to identify at operation (an aortotomy gives but limited access to the problem) and are therefore hard to extirpate.

The most useful aids to complete diagnosis in the post-mortem room are a detailed knowledge of cardiac anatomy coupled with a high degree of suspicion! The aortic and mitral valves are the most commonly involved in infective endocarditis; the tricuspid and pulmonary ones less so, except in the case of intravenous drug takers when the tricuspid valve is the most likely to be affected. In acute endocarditis the heart may have a soft, flabby texture and sometimes appears pale. As stated in Chapter 1, fixing the heart at least partially before beginning the dissection overcomes the problem of the soft texture.

Anatomy of the aortic root

Although infection of the aortic root accounts for only a small proportion of cases of infective endocarditis, it exemplifies to a marked degree the difficulties indicated in the preceding paragraphs. Because of its relative complexity, the anatomy is described in detail.

The aortic root comprises the three leaflets of the aortic valve and their respective aortic sinuses, the annulus fibrosus of the aortic valve, the membranous part of the ventricular septum, the infundibular septum, the area of aortomitral continuity and that part of the anterior leaflet of the mitral valve with which it is confluent. It is related to the transverse sinus of the pericardium by way of the posterior (non-coronary) and left aortic sinuses and the aortomitral fibrous continuity, which also permits potential communication with the left atrium. It is also related to the left atrium via the anterior mitral leaflet and to the left ventricle by means of the aortic leaflets. The aortic root is also related to the right atrium by the ventriculoatrial portion of the membranous septum, to the inlet part of the right ventricle by the interventricular portion of the membranous septum, and to the right ventricular outflow tract via the infundibular septum. The aortic root is therefore related to, and has potential connection with, all the chambers of the heart, as well as the pericardial cavity[2]. Both the posterior and left aortic leaflets and their sinuses arise from fibrous tissue (the membranous part of the ventricular septum and the area of aortomitral continuity, with which it is continuous).

Only the right sinus and leaflet are bedded in muscle (the infundibular septum), so that most of the aortic root is fibrous[2]. If this fibrous area is attacked by endocarditis, mycotic aneurysms, sometimes of enormous size, can develop and may rupture either inside or outside the heart[3]. By contrast, when the smaller, muscular part of the aortic root is affected, the right side of the heart may become involved. Aneurysms of the membranous septum occur with some frequency, and if they rupture they produce an interventricular communication. Even if this is haemodynamically quite insignificant, large areas of myocardium can become necrotic when the right side of the heart is involved as well. The valve lesions, not intracardiac shunts, are the usual culprits when there is grave haemodynamic derangement.

The membranous part of the ventricular septum is confluent with the inlet septum, which extends posteriorly to the crux cordis, and also with the muscular atrioventricular septum[2,4]. If this musculature becomes necrotic as a result of sepsis, cardiac rupture may occur. Less instantly catastrophic, the aortic valve and the left ventricle may become detached from one another. This event is called aortoventricular dissociation and can also occur when the fibrous components of the aortic root are also involved.

Perhaps rather remarkably, aortoventricular dissociation is a potentially recoverable surgical condition; septic cardiac rupture is not.

Infective endocarditis has a poor prognosis: the 5-year survival for all forms is 60%, while that for PVE is 50% at 6 months[5].

The specialized conducting system

The atrioventricular node is situated at the apex of the triangle (of Koch) formed by the valve of the coronary sinus (the thebesian valve), the 'annulus' of the tricuspid valve (which, unlike the mitral valve, does not possess a complete annulus fibrosus), and the membranous part of the ventricular septum. The common (undivided) bundle emerges from the node and immediately passes, in the central fibrous body (of which the annulus of the aortic valve is a part) to the ventricular aspect of the tricuspid 'ring', where it descends for a short distance to the inferior margin of the membranous septum. Here, the bundle bifurcates, the right branch continuing along the inferior rim of the membranous septum, soon to pass to the moderator band, while the left bundle branch takes origin from the right and passes over the summit of the muscular septum, beneath the membranous septum, to sweep down the smooth left ventricular aspect of the muscular septum, where it bifurcates into anterior and posterior fasciculi.

From the foregoing short account it is evident that the proximal part of the conducting system is intimately related to the membranous part of the ventricular septum and hence to the aortic root, so that it is likely to be involved in a septic process affecting the root. It is usually possible to demonstrate this microscopically with one or two sections; detailed studies of the cardiac conducting system involving serial sections are seldom necessary in this condition.

Atrioventricular valves

Where infection of a prosthetic atrioventricular valve is known or suspected the following are anticipated findings:

1. Paraprosthetic leak(s).
2. Immobilization of the prosthesis by thrombus.
3. Encroachment of pannus from the sewing ring.
4. Failure of the prosthesis to heal.
5. Vegetations (uncommon on mechanical valves).
6. Foci of calcification (sewing ring of mechanical valves).
7. Leaflet calcification (bioprostheses, but note that these calcify rapidly in juveniles without infection, thus their use is contraindicated in children and teenagers).
8. Mycotic aneurysms.
9. Septic emboli.
10. Myocardial abscesses.

The last three are less common findings.

The simplest means of identifying the features listed is to fix the heart before examining the valve area. The apex may, of course, be sectioned in the fresh state if preferred, after removal of such samples as may be needed for culture. It is advisable to inspect the coronary arteries for emboli (both visually and by gentle palpation), prior to fixation. If emboli are suspected, fixation by perfusion is not recommended. Loose blood may be washed out gently with water through fairly short incisions in the atria (Chapter 1) before immersion in the chosen fixative.

Enlarge the atrial incision fully to display the prosthesis. If there are no obvious paraprosthetic leaks (and they are usually fairly easy to see), probe the edge of the sewing ring. This often reveals further small cavities. If the sutures are still visible, gentle traction may demonstrate loose or pulled-out stitches. Repeat these procedures from the ventricular aspect of the valve before removing the prosthesis. This should be done in as close an approximation to the manner in which it was inserted as is feasible. If the valve was placed with continuous suture it requires only one or two snips on the atrial side to give sufficient length simply to pull it out. If, as is more usual, it was placed with interrupted stitches, it may be a little more difficult. Aim to preserve the native annulus rather than the prosthesis, as there may be numerous, small, undetected or unsuspected abscesses in the surrounding area. Generally the sutures are easy to see in PVE. Hold the knot end firmly with non-toothed forceps and, using small (preferably curved, round-ended) scissors, cut the suture below the knot. As the sutures are always double, this manoeuvre releases only one side of the stitch. The other is in the native annulus and must be freed by cautious use of the scissors curving towards the prosthesis.

It is rather easier to free all the valve sutures first, then proceed with removing those in the annulus. Cavities tunnelling into the myocardium may now be disclosed and evaluated, and calcified myocardial abscesses become easier to locate.

If there is an aortic valve *in situ* the process must be repeated. Mechanical aortic prostheses are more difficult to examine than tissue valves as, because of the poppet, it is generally impossible to pass either a probe or a sharp instrument to release the valve through the orifice.

If there are both aortic and mitral prostheses the aortic root is obligatorily distorted to a variable degree and the valves may have to be removed before a clear field of vision can be obtained. Aortic prostheses are taken out in the same way as mitral ones, but it is usually rather more difficult and requires patience.

If there are no obvious abscesses, etc., but they are suspected, the whole of the aortic root may be displayed by taking a 'ham-knife' and positioning the heart so that the cut will bisect the membranous septum. Take a single slice obliquely through the base of the heart so that half the specimen shows the ventricles and their valves (or where the valves have just been removed) while the other half has the aortic valve, the atria and part of the membranous septum (Figure 4.1). This procedure benefits from being practised beforehand if the prosector is less than perfectly acquainted with the fairly complex anatomy of the aortic root.

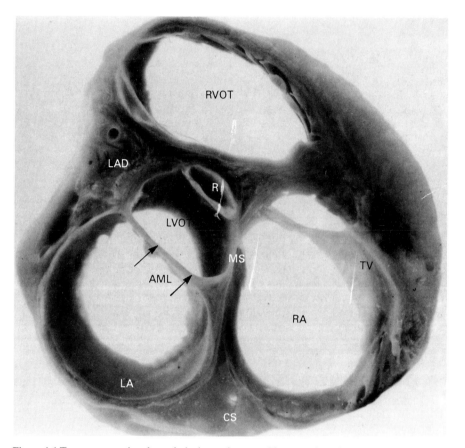

Figure 4.1 Transverse section through the base of a normal heart to show the aortic root and its relations. Only the right aortic leaflet (R) is bedded entirely in muscle; it lies slightly superior to the non-coronary and left aortic leaflets. Most of the left ventricular outflow tract (LVOT) is fibrous, consisting of the anterior mitral leaflet (AML, arrowed) and the membranous septum (MS). The anterior descending branch of the left coronary artery (LAD) passes through muscle in this heart, rather than taking the more usual epicardial course. CS, coronary sinus; LA, left atrium; RA, right atrium; RVOT, right ventricular outflow tract; TV, tricuspid valve

The coronary arteries do not generally demonstrate features peculiar to PVE, but meticulous sectioning will, of course, reveal any septic emboli. Mycotic aneurysms are not usually difficult to identify, while intraluminal disease occurs in older patients with the same frequency as in non-infected patients.

The apparent timelessness of late PVE is remarkable. Even when the attack of infective endocarditis was many years ago there may be large, deep and still increasing abscess cavities (Figure 4.2). It is often possible to obtain positive Gram stains from such tissues, even years after the patient was supposedly cured of the infection.

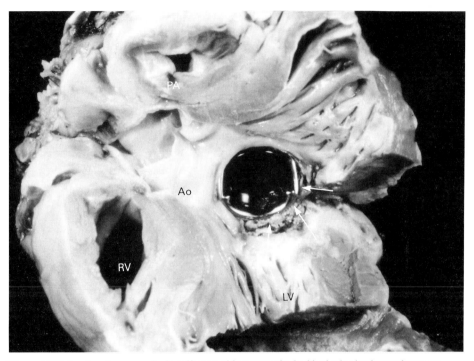

Figure 4.2 Extensive abscess cavity in a 60-year-old women who had had mitral valve replacement (Bjork–Shiley valve) 5 years previously and had supposedly recovered from prosthetic valve endocarditis 3 years before she died, following reoperation. The cavity (arrowed) extends posteriorly from the area of aortomitral continuity to the obtuse margin of the heart so that it occupies about a third of the annulus. Ao, aortic valve; PA, pulmonary artery; LV, left ventricle; RV, right ventricle

Septic myocarditis is an anticipated finding in severe infections and extensive myocardial necrosis can result. Additionally, discrete myocardial abscesses are a relatively common finding and these may calcify once they have healed. The simplest means of locating them is by a penetrated X-ray, for, like calcified plaque in coronary arteries, they can cause severe damage to the knife during gross examination, with the potential for injury to the prosector.

References

1. Westaby, S., Oakley, C. M., Sapsford, R. N. and Bentall, H. H. Surgical treatment of infective endocarditis with special reference to prosthetic valve endocarditis. *British Medical Journal,* **287**, 320–323, 1983

2. Allwork, S. P. The anatomical basis of infection of the aortic root. *Thoracic and Cardiovascular Surgeon,* **34**, 143–148, 1986
3. McManus, B. M., Katz, N. M., Blackbourne, B. D. *et al.* Acquired cor triatriatum (left ventricular false aneurysm): complication of active infective endocarditis of the aortic valve with ring abscess treated by aortic valve replacement. *American Heart Journal,* **104,** 312–314, 1982
4. Allwork, S. P. Anatomical versus embryological nomenclature in cardiac malformations exemplified by interatrial communications. *Theoretical Surgery,* **2**, 129–132, 1987
5. Durack, D. Prosthetic valve endocarditis. In *Aspects of Infection. No. 1: Management Strategies in Infective Endocarditis* (ed. R. Stepney), Eli Lilly, Basingstoke, UK, p. 3.2, 1987

5

Myocardial revascularization

Although bypass grafting is currently the most common surgical treatment for coronary artery disease, it is increasingly being replaced by angioplasty techniques. These may be performed either percutaneously or under direct vision at surgical operation.

Percutaneous transluminal coronary angioplasty (PTCA) is a little outside the scope of this book, except insofar as complications during the procedure may necessitate emergency bypass grafting (for example, if an acute dissection of a coronary artery occurs). PTCA can take as long as a bypass operation ($2\frac{1}{2}$–3 h), and complications requiring surgical treatment, while not common, are not unknown. An excellent account of the pathological findings after repeated PTCA is given by Ueda *et al.* [1].

Laser angioplasty is in its infancy; at present the laser is used as a sophisticated cautery rather than as a light beam. In early death following laser angioplasty the surrounding area is oedematous and may be haemorrhagic. The artery itself may be punctured (this was a complication in the earliest work, when the laser beam hit the nearest bend in an artery), but it is uncommon now as modifications to the tip of the fibreoptic disperse the beam. The more usual finding is a variable degree of thermal injury, ranging from microscopically detectable to frank charring readily recognized with the naked eye. The surrounding tissue granulates after a few days.

Anatomy and nomenclature of the coronary arteries

The following terminology is used in surgical anatomy of the coronary arteries.

Right coronary artery

The right coronary artery originates in the right (anteromedial) aortic sinus and soon gives an infundibular branch (not amenable to grafting), which passes anteriorly to the pulmonary infundibulum. This branch commonly anastomoses with a small branch of the left coronary artery to form the anastomotic ring (of Vieussens). These branches and the ring are sometimes very considerably enlarged in disease.

The second branch passes to the atrium, where, in about 55% of people, it eventually vascularizes the sinuatrial node. The right coronary artery passes in the right atrioventricular sulcus to the acute margin of the heart, giving a variable number of right ventricular branches (again not grafted). At the acute margin there is a fairly constant branch, the acute marginal branch, which is sometimes grafted (Figure 5.1).

The right artery usually continues in the atrioventricular sulcus until the crux of the heart is reached. Here it loops into the myocardium; a small branch passes to the atrioventricular node in most individuals, and the main artery divides into a posterior descending branch, which is a most important vessel for grafting, and a posterolateral branch which crosses the posterior interventricular sulcus to terminate as the posterolateral branch, which is also often grafted. Less commonly, the vital posterior descending branch originates at the acute margin to pass obliquely across it and gain the posterior interventricular sulcus.

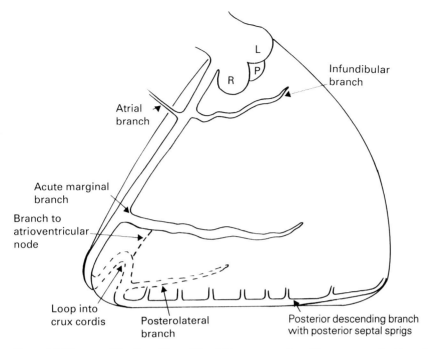

Figure 5.1 Diagram of the disposition of the right coronary artery. The acute marginal branch is a fairly constant feature and the loop into the myocardium at the crux cordis is seen in a right anterior oblique projection. L, left aortic valve leaflet; R, right aortic valve leaflet; P, posterior aortic valve leaflet

Left coronary artery

The left coronary artery originates in the left (anterolateral) aortic sinus and passes undivided for up to 2.5 cm as the *left main coronary artery*. It generally bifurcates into *anterior descending* and *circumflex branches*, but in about a third of individuals it trifurcates. The branch between the anterior descending and circumflex branches is called the *intermediate branch (ramus intermedius)* (Figure 5.2).

The anterior descending branch passes in the anterior interventricular sulcus towards the apex. During its course it gives a variable number of branches (*diagonal branches*) to the left ventricle. These, together with their parent branch, are important for grafting. The first diagonal branch is a major vessel which originates in the proximal third of the anterior descending branch. It may reach the apex of the heart, and is quite often submerged in muscle for part of its length. When the left coronary artery trifurcates this first diagonal branch is replaced by the intermediate branch. In addition to the diagonal branches passing to the left ventricle, there are smaller (not grafted) branches passing to the right ventricle, as described above (Figure 5.3).

In addition to the diagonal and right ventricular sprigs, the anterior descending branch of the left coronary artery also gives a number of branches passing from its underside (epicardial aspect), vertically downwards into the anterior ventricular septum. These important arterial branches are the *septal branches*, sometimes also called the septal perforators or perforating branches. They are variable in number

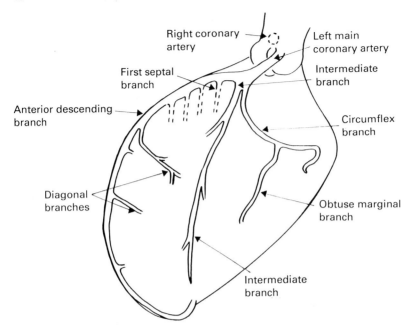

Figure 5.2 Diagram to show trifurcation of the left coronary artery into anterior descending, intermediate and circumflex branches. When present, an intermediate branch replaces significant diagonal branches in most people

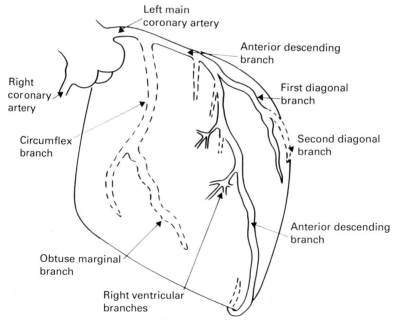

Figure 5.3 Diagram of the left coronary artery and its branches. Sprigs pass to the right from the anterior descending branch and may be distinguished from septal branches by their angle of origin

and site of origin, except for the first branch. The 'first septal' artery is a relatively large branch (1–2 mm in diameter in normal people) which takes origin from the anterior descending branch close to the origin of the first diagonal branch (see Figure 5.2). This branch can become greatly enlarged in coronary artery disease and may be difficult to distinguish angiographically from other branches unless several projections are examined.

The posterior descending branch, whether from the left or the right coronary artery, also gives septal branches; although they are smaller than those vascularizing the anterior septum, they are no less important. Much myocardium may be lost if the posterior descending branch is occluded.

The circumflex branch of the left coronary artery occupies the left atrioventricular sulcus and gives a variable number of branches called *obtuse marginal branches*, which are grafted. The circumflex artery itself is not graftable because of its inaccessibility in the left atrioventricular groove. In 70% of people the circumflex branch terminates as an obtuse marginal branch at or near the obtuse margin of the heart (see Figure 5.2).

The foregoing describes the anatomy to be found in the majority of people (i.e. that the artery supplying the posterior descending branch is the right coronary artery). This arrangement is called right coronary dominance. Although the left coronary artery always supplies a greater mass of muscle than does the right, it is not usually dominant. Left dominance (posterior descending branch is the continuation of the circumflex) is found in only about 15% of people [2,3].

Detailed, illustrated accounts of the numerous variants of coronary anatomy and their significance are given elsewhere, together with the morphology and significance of both the coronary and non-coronary collateral blood supply to the heart [3–7].

Bypass grafts

It is helpful to know in advance of the necropsy whether the patient had internal thoracic artery grafts as well as saphenous vein grafts, as the former may be damaged irrevocably if the body is opened without due regard to them. The absence of leg wounds obviously identifies patients who had only arterial or other sorts of graft, but their presence does not preclude the use of other kinds of graft (see Chapter 1).

If the long saphenous veins are unavailable (previous operation) or unsuitable (severe varices), arm veins or man-made grafts or, less commonly, bioprostheses in the form of umbilical veins are utilized instead. The internal thoracic artery (usually called the internal mammary artery) is increasingly being used for the left coronary artery and its branches, as the long-term patency is better than that of veins. (This procedure should not be confused with the long-obsolete operation of Vineberg, in which the internal thoracic (internal mammary) artery was implanted directly into the myocardium with the object of stimulating the collateral circulation [8].) The internal thoracic artery is more often used in men; it tends to be rather small in women, with consequent poor flow.

There are several complications which may be associated with these internal mammary arteries. The dissection at operation to collect the artery may cause much bleeding, especially in fat people, and many surgeons consider obesity to be a contraindication to the procedure for this reason. Similarly, the dissection can give rise to sepsis, especially in the old, so that age (over about 70 years) may also be considered to be a contraindication. Some surgeons measure the flow through the artery before implanting it and discard it if the flow is poor. Thus the patient has had all the disadvantages of having the artery prepared for grafting, without the benefits of an arterial graft. (Poor flow is often associated with arterial spasm during dissection; this is largely overcome by manoeuvres such as wrapping the graft in a swab moistened with papaverine to lessen the spasm.)

Although the left internal mammary artery is used for up to three-quarters of all grafts to the left anterior descending branch, internal mammary artery grafts account for only about one-quarter of all the bypass grafts done in the UK, so that vein grafts still constitute most of the surgical cases.

Vein grafts

Irrespective of their source, vein grafts are often abbreviated to ACABG (aortocoronary bypass grafts) or CABG (coronary artery bypass grafts). Less commonly, the term CVG (coronary vein grafts) is used. This last is most unsatisfactory, as the coronary veins are not concerned at all. (As a matter of purely historical interest, however, there was once an operation in which the coronary sinus, the debouchment of most of the coronary veins, was connected to the aorta so that there was, in theory, retrograde perfusion of the coronary arteries.)

Vein grafts are anastomosed into the ascending aorta singly, but sometimes quite close to each other. A separate stoma is made for each one. The anastomoses are made with continuous suture and generally cause no problems with bleeding.

The distal anastomoses vary a little. They may be applied singly to a coronary branch, in which case the vein is tailored so that the anastomosis is slightly enlarged end-to-side. Alternatively, a longer length of vein may be used for sequential anastomoses, known as 'snake', 'sequential' or 'horseshoe' grafts; in these, the anastomoses are made side-to-side. Grafts to the obtuse marginal branches are often passed through the transverse sinus of the pericardium to reach their destination. This manoeuvre has a threefold advantage: it reduces the risk of compression when the chest is closed, the shorter length of vein has better flow and it saves vein. The circumflex branch itself is not grafted directly, due to its inaccessibility in the left atrioventricular sulcus.

The distal anastomoses, like the proximal ones, are made with a fine (6/0 or less) monofilament suture. As they are usually done with the aid of a magnifying loup the suture lines seldom leak (see below).

Concomitant procedures

Endarterectomy   The distal right coronary artery may be prepared for grafting by this means; the left system is less amenable to it. Removal of a cast of plaque may damage the arterial wall, particularly if there is calcification, and dissection or early postoperative occlusion may result.

Ventricular aneurysmectomy   This may be performed at the time of grafting, the wound is closed in two layers, usually with continuous suture.

Valve replacement   Calcific aortic valve stenosis coexists with some frequency, particularly in the over-70s. Replacement adds but little to the risk[9]. As some patients with rheumatic or other valve disease have concomitant coronary artery disease, atrioventricular valve replacement may be done at the same time.

Closure of ischaemic septal rupture   Surgical closure of ischaemic ventricular septal defect (VSD) is increasingly being done in the acute phase. The defects are quite unlike congenital VSDs; they are usually multiple, among the apical trabeculae and irregularly shaped. There is usually no distinct morphology, the defects consisting only of perforations due to necrosis. Closure is effected by direct suture, usually over pledgets of felt or similar material. The operation is often combined with excision of a ventricular aneurysm so that there may not be a separate ventriculotomy for the VSD closure.

In these patients, with manifestly poor myocardial function, the haemodynamic derangement caused by the sudden left-to-right shunt in the presence of low cardiac output may be the prime contributor to death. A frequent finding is occlusion of the proximal part of the posterior descending coronary artery in individuals with poor or absent collateral circulation. Thus, people with dominant left coronary artery are especially at risk, as are those with previous anterolateral or apical infarction.

Assessment of the repair can be done through an incision parallel to the ventriculotomy. At first sight there may be little to see from the right ventricle, as the rupture is usually a breakdown of the trabeculae carneae posteriorly. Probing will often indicate the site of repair(s), which is often easier to see from the left ventricle. If the surgical incision did not include the left ventricle, it will be necessary to open this chamber with the probe *in situ*.

Abolition of arrythmia   Surgical treatment of this complication of myocardial infarction may utilize cryoablation, cautery, resection or encircling ventriculotomy from within the chamber.

The site of cryoablation is difficult to identify unless it was marked at the operation by a suture. It appears as a lesion of 1 cm diameter or less, and looks like an infarction.

Encircling ventriculotomy is made using either cautery or a knife. In the latter case the resulting wound is sutured. The chamber can be approached either through an aneurysm, when present, or through the aortic valve, or via a short, full-thickness ventriculotomy.

Early death

The most common causes of death early in the postoperative period are:

1. Persistent low cardiac output.
2. Cardiogenic shock.
3. Evolving myocardial infarction.
4. Perioperative myocardial infarction.
5. Technical problems associated with the operation.

Technical problems either cause myocardial infarction or fail to improve the blood supply to a heart already critically ischaemic. Factors complicating the collection of internal mammary arteries are outlined above. Overlong grafts can kink, cutting off the flow. The grafts may be compressed by the sternum or, rarely, by a chest drain. This is not easy to identify in the post-mortem room as the chest drain has invariably been taken out before the body arrives, but it may have left its impression on the surrounding tissues. The veins themselves may accidentally have been narrowed during ligation of the tributaries, causing poor 'run-off' to the downstream myocardium.

Examination of the heart

While it is better to begin the study on the unfixed heart (it is easier to see and date the infarction), care is needed to avoid damaging the distal anastomoses. Pericardial adhesion begins early and it is disappointingly easy to avulse a graft by stripping the pericardium off. Although time consuming, it is better to use blunt dissection (the fingers are particularly useful here).

It is helpful to have available some means of magnification for the distal anastomoses. Even an ordinary magnifying glass will suffice, but the task is made much easier if an illuminated magnifying glass is available.

Patency of the grafts can be confirmed quite simply. When fully patent they are, of course, flat. The presence of ante-mortem thrombus indicates poor run-off and usually points to new infarction (the tissue surrounding the native artery is literally 'stuffed' with blood) immediately distal to the anastomosis. If this area is examined by sectioning it transversely, beginning at the anastomosis, it will usually reveal that the distal artery is either very small or that there is diffuse disease which had not been demonstrable by preoperative angiography. This, and prolonged periods of low-output failure permitting stasis, are the only real causes of non-patent grafts in the early postoperative period. The technical problems outlined above are very uncommon, as coronary grafting, particularly with veins, is such an oft-perfomed operation.

When death occurs 7–10 days after operation a broader spectrum of findings may be anticipated.

Tamponade

This may be due to ventricular rupture subsequent to preoperative or perioperative infarction. (While in 'medical' patients confirmation of the diagnosis of infarction generally presents no difficulties, virtually none of the diagnostic criteria, e.g. enzymes, ECG changes, are reliable in patients who have just undergone operations under cardiopulmonary bypass.)

An uncommon cause of tamponade is a *leaking false aneurysm* due to a suture cutting out of a distal anastomosis (Figure 5.4). Graft disruption due to overwhelming infection is a very rare event.

Myocardial necrosis

Foci of necrosis are always demonstrable after cardiopulmonary bypass, irrespective of discrete infarction[10]. Large areas of myocardium are susceptible if cardiac output is low for prolonged periods. If the operation included closure of a VSD, a degree of breakdown of the closure can result from spreading necrosis, despite the most meticulous attention to excision of necrotic myocardium at operation. Ischaemic VSDs are usually located posteroapically, among the trabeculae, so that it is not uncommon to find probe patencies. These are usually

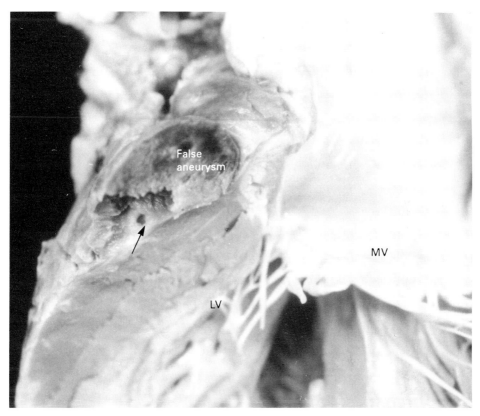

Figure 5.4 Leaking suture line anastomosing a vein graft to the first diagonal branch of the left coronary artery. The pinhole leak (arrow) caused a large false aneurysm. The patient's postoperative course lasted 3 weeks and had been stormy, with recurrent episodes of hypotension. LV, left ventricle; MV, mitral valve

haemodynamically insignificant, particularly as cardiac output tends to have been low in these patients.

Myocardial infarction
Infarction in the immediate preoperative period is an increasing indication for emergency operation, so that death at a week or so is relatively common too, despite urgent revascularization of the heart. The same applies to perioperative infarction and to those occurring early in the postoperative period, when they are difficult to confirm by the usual means.

It is difficult to identify myocardial necrosis of less than 6 h duration, but dead myocytes (stained with haematoxylin and eosin) fluoresce when examined in ultraviolet light[10] and will fluoresce even in unstained material. This phenomenon occurs immediately, as the edges of a myocardial biopsy will show, and is independent of autolysis and long-term storage.

Myocardial necrosis can be demonstrated by a number of techniques, including staining of slices of fresh tissue with nitro-blue tetrazolium. Unaffected tissue takes up the stain, and is uniformly blue, while dead myocardium is unstained, due to loss of mitochondrial dehydrogenase in the dead fibres. Fibrous tissue appears white.

Dead myocardial fibres are fuchsinophilic for about 12 h after death, and a number of special stains based on both acid and basic fuchsin are available. They all have the disadvantage of technical complexity and are indiscriminate, in that myocytes dead from any cause, e.g. anoxia, are stained, especially in the subendocardium.

After about 8 h, microscopic morphological changes are discernible without special stains, beginning with pyknosis of the nuclei and swelling of the mitochondria, while macroscopic changes, beginning with the appearance of a haemorrhagic area, are evident after about 12 h.

Discrimination between regional and diffuse necrosis in the early postoperative period may be possible by identifying the timing of the progress of the necrotic lesion. Diffuse necrosis is a fairly common finding in patients with previous low cardiac output, but regional necrosis will be confined to the area supplied by the coronary artery branch involved in the procedure.

Complications associated with valve replacement

Aortic valve replacement is seldom implicated, but left ventricular rupture associated with a mitral valve replacement may be (see Chapter 3). Most patients who need mitral valve replacement for ischaemic mitral regurgitation have left ventricles more or less normal thickness (unless they are severely hypertensive) so that the risk of rupture is increased when ischaemic or infarcted papillary muscles are involved.

It is usually difficult to distinguish grossly between left ventricular rupture due to papillary muscle necrosis and that consequent upon preoperative or perioperative infarction. Microscopy sometimes helps, but as the events causing the necrosis tend to be more or less contemporaneous, especially when the procedure was done as an emergency, it is not infallible.

Late death

Myocardial revascularization is an atypical form of surgical therapy in that, although it abolishes the symptoms in the majority of patients, it neither cures nor arrests the underlying disease. Thus, patients who die late after operation (which can be repeated a number of times to relieve symptoms) may or may not have non-patency of one or all of the grafts, but they will have progression of the underlying disease.

As there are so many people with bypass grafts the causes of late death among them are legion, but ischaemic heart disease is probably the most common and is likely to be implicated in the others.

Graft failure

Late graft failure is associated with healing of the graft itself, in that occlusion is often due to exaggerated healing. When the vein is removed from the leg it loses much of its adventitia and it is exposed to arterial blood pressure. As a consequence, the intimal endothelium, deprived of its blood supply from its vasa vasorum, is lost as well. The changes which take place to repair this damage initiate the process of healing. The loss of the endothelium produces oedema and a transient, acute inflammatory cell reaction in the intima and subjacent media. Microthrombi and fibrin are deposited on the intima, and these, together with proliferating smooth muscle cells, fibroblasts and endothelial cells, form a new, pseudointima by the end of 4–6 weeks. This new surface reaches its maximal thickness after 4–6 months. During the ensuing 6 months the new surface condenses and fibroses. The media also loses its blood supply at transplantation from the leg, so that many smooth muscle cells die and are replaced by fibrous tissue. The surviving myocytes hypertrophy, causing the media to become relatively thick and firm. The adventitia is replaced by scar tissue which eventually revascularizes; by the end of a year the graft is arterialized, i.e. it has a firm, thickened wall and a patent lumen.

The 'healed' graft may have a lumen lined with mature fibrous tissue covered by endothelium. This is called a neointima, but the lumen may be lined with other material, for example fibrin and/or collagen. When this happens, the lining is a pseudointima. Smooth muscle cells acquire some of the characteristics of endothelial cells when they are exposed to a bloodstream, so that positive identification of a neointima depends on identifying some product of endothelial cells, e.g. factor VIII, before naming the new inner capsule[11].

It is the nature of the new lining which may be problematical with respect to graft failure. Slight graft–artery mismatch can cause jet lesions (see Chapter 4) close to the anastomosis, but much more commonly there is exaggerated fibrosis of the new intimal layer, which is often concentric. This condition is called *fibrointimal hyperplasia* and may continue to develop until the lumen of the graft is occluded.

The foregoing readily explains the superior patency rate of internal thoracic artery grafts, but these too may develop the changes described, although usually to a much lesser degree. Other materials used for aortocoronary grafts usually develop a pseudointima, but man, in contrast to some other species, has little ability to heal long lengths or large areas of prosthetic material. True healing, with development of a neointima, occurs only at and close to the anastomoses[12].

It has been stated that up to a third of patients have stenoses in their grafts by the end of the first year. The factors governing this are multifactorial[13]. Thrombosis is a rare cause of late graft failure and becomes more so the longer the patient survives. Most thrombotic occlusions of the graft occur within the first postoperative year[14]. Graft occlusion is due either to progressive intimal hyperplasia or to atheromatous disease progressing to the grafts[15]. Rarely, a slightly too-long graft, and therefore always slightly kinked, is 'suddenly' occluded by intimal hyperplasia. Patients who had endarterectomy at operation are especially affected, as the damaged arterial wall is stimulated by platelet activity to intimal hyperplasia.

A rare cause of graft failure, non-fatal in itself but likely to be contributory, is 'steal' phenomenon by a graft. Vein grafts become arterialized very quickly, and intimal proliferation, which is mediated by platelet activity, may also begin early (Figure 5.5). The underlying disease remains active and there is lipid turnover even in plaques covered by a fibrous cap[16], so that it is hardly surprising that the process affects the grafts sooner or later. The mechanisms whereby this occurs are uncertain, but probably have an anatomical basis, at least in part. The vasa vasorum of the coronary arteries communicate with the lumen and are dilated where there are plaques.

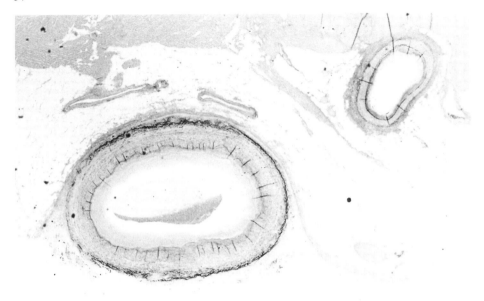

(a)

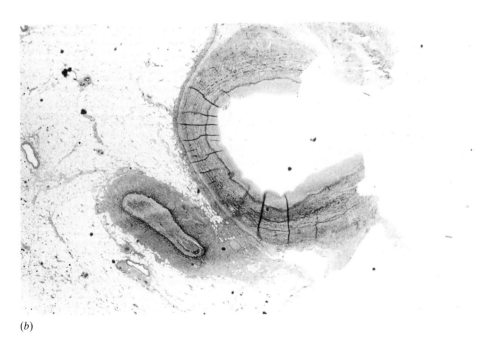

(b)

Figure 5.5 60-year-old man who died suddenly in pulmonary oedema. (a) Arterialized distal part of a graft to the anterior descending branch of the left coronary artery 8 weeks after operation. (b) Graft to the right coronary artery (opened longitudinally) is also arterialized and shows marked intimal proliferation. (Elastic van Gieson, ×6)

Examination of the heart

Although it is appreciated that it will usually be impossible, study of the most recent postoperative coronary arteriograms is the ideal aid to the examination of the heart, as they identify the location of the grafts. Although the grafts are often very difficult to see, particularly the right, they may be palpable. It is helpful to try to locate them by palpation before removing the pericardium, as considerable damage to them can result from the sharp dissection which is often necessary for this manoeuvre.

Because of early arterialization and the almost inevitable intimal hyperplasia, the grafts feel firm to the touch, even when widely patent. That to the right coronary artery is often invisible as it quickly becomes buried in fat in the right atrioventricular sulcus so that it resembles a native artery. Those to the anterior branches of the left system are usually visible and resemble large, firm native arteries. Grafts passing through the transverse sinus, like those to the right, are invisible for much of their length.

The proximal ends of the grafts are, fortunately, usually easy to see, so that, if necessary, the graft can be traced from its origin.

In the case of vein grafts, early occlusion causes the vein to atrophy, so that it may be impossible to locate on the heart. Sometimes the surgeon places a radio-opaque marker at the aortic end to facilitate postoperative arteriography, and this may be a clue to the site of the graft. The tributaries of the vein are ligated with thread, and their remnants sometimes identify the site.

Internal thoracic artery grafts also fail and atrophy, in which case they are impossible to find unless there are still either a few suture ends visible from the anastomosis or the metal clips used to ligate the branches of the artery can be found.

In late deaths, the occlusion, if present or suspected, is not usually at the site of the distal anastomosis, so that meticulous cleaning of that part is usually unnecessary. The occlusion can be found more easily if the angiogram or the report is available.

The grafts can be sectioned either longitudinally or transversely (the latter enables better assessment of the patency but longitudinal section keeps the specimen together, particularly if the grafts are not firmly adherent to the epicardial surface).

Collateral circulation

When the grafts are atheromatous the native arteries proximal to them are often totally occluded. The distal segments of the vessels show advanced disease and may themselves be occluded. If the collateral vessels fed by the graft are epicardial, it is sometimes possible to recognize them with the naked eye. Most collateral channels are intramuscular and are recognized as numerous small (0.5–0.75 mm) vessels in the cut surface of the left ventricle. They appear microscopically as small muscular arteries which pass obliquely through the muscle fibres and are unaccompanied by veins or nerves.

In addition to these coronary collateral arteries, there may also be collateral vessels which are non-coronary in origin. These appear as small, tortuous vessels entering the pericardium, both along the great arteries and veins and through the pericardial reflections. These vessels originate from the vasa vasorum of the great vessels and from the bronchial, pericardial and mediastinal vasculature. They pass mainly to the atria, where they anastomose with the atrial arteries, and although their flow is very small, (up to 12 ml/min/100 g in the atria and 0.75 ml/min/100 g in the ventricles) it may account for the curious condition in which reasonably good left ventricular function is maintained in individuals whose coronary arteries appear totally occluded at angiography[7,17].

Although there is a wealth of literature on the collateral circulation, the factors which influence its reopening or development are as yet incompletely understood. Collateral vessels are not present in all ischaemic hearts but, when they are, they are recognizable at necropsy.

Myocardial infarction

Recent infarction and its sequelae are obviously anticipated findings at necropsy in these patients, particularly when there is graft failure. Even in patients grafted with no history of infarction there is usually extensive myocardial fibrosis. This is not confined to the most hypertensive patients.

Infective endocarditis

Patients who have had revascularization operations without other procedures are not especially susceptible to endocarditis (see Table 4.1). If there are prosthetic valves as well, the risks of endocarditis are the same as those of valve replacement alone.

Arrythmias

As mentioned above, the site of arrythmias treated by cryoablation is almost impossible to find either early or late, unless it was marked at the time of operation. The cryoprobe makes a lesion about 1 cm in diameter and up to 5 mm deep. The thermal injury is confined to this size, and although it results in necrosis, this does not spread as it does in coagulation necrosis due to ischaemia[18]. The lesion heals to a small scar. Ablation of an arrythmic focus using cautery also causes thermal damage and heals in the same way as the cold burns, but leaves a slightly larger scar. Encircling ventriculotomy heals to a thin raised scar; sutures may still be visible.

References

1. Ueda, M., Becker, A. E. and Fujimoto, T. Pathological changes induced by repeated percutaneous transluminal coronary angioplasty. *British Heart Journal,* **58**, 635–643, 1987
2. Allwork, S. P. Angiographic anatomy. In *Cardiac Anatomy* (eds R. H. Anderson and A. E. Becker), Gower, London, Chapter 7, 1980
3. Allwork, S. P. and Raphael, M. J. Patterns of coronary artery distribution: radiological and anatomical correlations. In *Cardiovascular Surgery* (eds W. Bircks, J. Ostermeyer and H. D. Schulte), Springer Verlag, Heidelberg, pp. 196–199, 1980
4. Raphael, M. J., Hawtin, D. R. and Allwork, S. P. The angiographic anatomy of the coronary arteries. *British Journal of Surgery,* **67**, 181–187, 1980
5. Allwork, S. P. A spectrum of normal coronary artery distribution in man. *Anatomia Clinica,* **1**, 311–319, 1979
6. Allwork, S. P. The anatomy of the coronary arteries. In *The Surgery of Coronary Artery Disease* (ed. D. J. Wheatley), Chapman and Hall, London, pp. 15–25, 1986
7. Allwork, S. P. The applied anatomy of the arterial blood supply to the heart in man. *Journal of Anatomy,* **153**, 1–16, 1987

8. Vineberg, A. M. Development of an anastomosis between the coronary vessels and a transplanted internal mammary artery. *Canadian Medical Association Journal,* **55,** 117–119, 1946

9. Nunley, D. Z., Grunkemeir, G. L. and Starr, A. Aortic valve replacement with coronary bypass grafting; significant determinants of 10 year survival. *Journal of Thoracic and Cardiovascular Surgery,* **85,** 705–711, 1983

10. Allwork, S. P. and Bentall, H. H. The usefulness of the phenomenon of histofluorescence in the identification of early myocardial necrosis. *Cardiovascular Research,* **20,** 451–457, 1986

11. Clowes, A. W., Collazzo, R. E. and Karnowsky, M. J. A morphologic and permeability study of luminal smooth muscle cells after arterial injury in the rat. *Laboratory Investigation,* **39,** 141–150, 1978

12. Clowes, A. W., Kirkman, T. R. and Reidy, M. A. Mechanisms of arterial graft healing. Rapid transmural capillary ingrowth provides a source of intimal endothelium and smooth muscle in porous PTFE prostheses. *American Journal of Pathology,* **123,** 220–230, 1986

13. Campeau, L., Enjalbert, M., Lesperance, J. *et al.* The relationship of risk factors to the development of atherosclerosis in saphenous vein bypass grafts and the progression of disease in the native circulation. *New England Journal of Medicine,* **311,** 1329–1332, 1984

14. Campeau, L., Crocker, D., Lesperance, J. *et al.* Postoperative changes in aortocoronary saphenous vein grafts revisited. Angiographic studies at 2 weeks and 1 year on 2 series of consecutive patients. *Circulation,* **52,** 369–377, 1975

15. Vladovar, Z. and Edwards, J. E. Pathologic changes in aortocoronary arterial saphenous grafts. *Circulation,* **44,** 719–728, 1971

16. Katz, S. S., Small, D. M., Smith, F. R. *et al.* Cholesterol turnover in lipid phases of human atherosclerotic plaque. *Journal of Lipid Research,* **23,** 733–737, 1982

17. Brazier, J., Hottenrott, C. and Buckberg, G. Noncoronary collateral myocardial blood flow. *Annals of Thoracic Surgery,* **19,** 426–435, 1977

18. Misaki, T., Allwork, S. P. and Bentall, H. H. Longterm effects of cryosurgery in the sheep heart. *Cardiovascular Research,* **17,** 61–69, 1983

6

Miscellaneous operations

Tumours of the heart

Primary cardiac tumours are rare[1,2]. Most large Units are unlikely to have more than about one case a year, and most of the tumours will be myxomata[3] but, of the malignant tumours, sarcoma predominates[4]. Cardiac metastases from malignant tumours are only very rarely treated surgically.

The surgical specimen obviously holds more interest for the pathologist than a heart from which the tumour has been removed! *Early death* following excision of a benign tumour is very uncommon and is more likely to be due to complications of cardiopulmonary bypass (see Chapter 1) than to the tumour itself.

In *late death* the heart is likely to be unremarkable. Although myxomata occasionally recur[5], they are as amenable to reoperation as to first operation.

Surgical ablation of arrythmia

Most patients whose arrythmias are treated surgically have ischaemic heart disease (see Chapter 5), but those with re-entrant arrythmias can have the accessory connection permanently abolished by a surgical operation.

Anatomical basis of re-entrant arrythmias

The specialized conducting system of the heart develops from 'rings' of primitive specialized tissue which surround the atrioventricular and ventriculoarterial junctions in the embryonic heart[6]. Islands of this ring tissue are found in all fetal hearts and in about 20% of adult hearts[7]. This was the tissue which Kent described in his series of papers on atrioventricular conduction at the turn of the century, and to which he attributed (incorrectly) normal atrioventricular conduction[8,9]. Although ring tissue can sometimes be found in the anticipated site of the connection (Figure 6.1), there is little evidence that this persistent fetal tissue is a source of pre-excitation in the adult; however, its presence explains the exasperating habit (particularly among surgeons) of referring to abnormal accessory atrioventricular connections, such as those often responsible for Wolff–Parkinson–White (WPW) syndrome, as 'Kent bundles'[10,11].

Accessory connections were first demonstrated in WPW syndrome in 1943[12]. They occur between both right atrium and ventricle (WPW type B) and left atrium and ventricle (WPW type A); the two are morphologically disimilar, due to the differences between the two atrioventricular annuli. It is stressed that accessory connections are usually no more than one or two cells wide, although they may be several cells long, so that they are very difficult to locate in the necropsy specimen unless one has access to the ECG, at the very least. The aid of the electrophysiologist is invaluable for these cases, as the connections can be located with great accuracy in living patients. The electrophysiological report greatly increases the chance of finding the connection at necropsy. Even with the results available, finding the connection may necessitate cutting several hundred serial sections without losing any. It is extremely laborious and time consuming but, if one succeeds in finding the fibre, an almost perfect clinicopathological correlation can be made. It is usually mandatory to divide the tissue block for histological

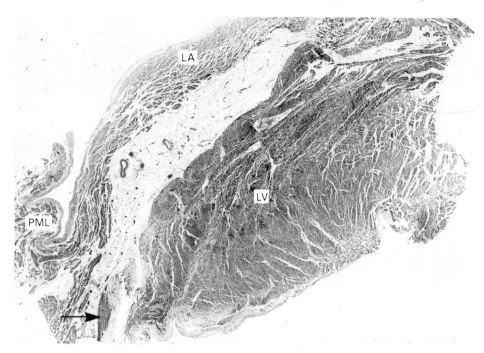

Figure 6.1 Ring tissue (arrowed) at the atrioventricular junction in a patient with WPW type A. Serial sectioning showed no accessory connections, but the ring tissue persisted for more than 200 μm. PML, medial scallop of the posterior mitral leaflet; LA, left atrium; LV, left ventricle. (Haematoxylin and eosin, ×6)

processing, automatically creating the potential for the loss of the critical one or two sections, but the cooperation of the electrophysiologist helps to minimize this very real risk.

Right-sided connections

The tricuspid valve normally has an incomplete annulus fibrosus, so that accessory connections can pass through the annulus, close to the valve (Figure 6.2). This anatomical fact is particularly well exemplified by the high incidence of WPW type B in Ebstein's anomaly of the tricuspid valve.

Left-sided connections

The mitral valve has a thick annulus fibrosus which completely encircles it to provide electrical insulation, *inter alia*, from the left atrium, so that accessory connections (WPW type A) must pass behind the annulus in the fat and connective tissues of the left atrioventricular sulcus. They may be quite superficial on the left side (Figure 6.3).

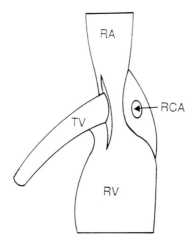

Figure 6.2 Diagram of the right atrioventricular junction. Because the tricuspid valve (TV) lacks a complete annulus fibrosus, right-sided accessory connections can pass through the annulus. RA, right atrium; RV, right ventricle; RCA, right coronary artery

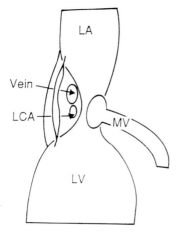

Figure 6.3 Diagram of the left atrioventricular junction. The mitral valve (MV) has a complete fibrous annulus insulating the ventricular myocardium from that of the atrium. Accessory connections must pass behind this fibrous tissue, and they may be placed quite superficially in the fat of the atrioventricular groove. LA, left atrium; LV, left ventricle; LCA, left coronary artery

Atrioventricular junction

A short account of this area is given, together with the connections associated with it, although arrythmias resulting from them are not usually amenable to operation other than ablation of the atrioventricular node itself. Clinical and operation notes are sometimes very confusing on this subject, due in no small part to the sometimes indiscriminate use of eponymous terms without much appreciation of their significance.

The atrioventricular node lies at the apex of the triangle of Koch, the inferior limb of which is formed by the posterior leaflet of the tricuspid valve, the posterior limb by the coronary sinus and the superior limb by the insertion of the tendinous extension of the eustachian (inferior vena cava) valve (called the tendon of Todaro) into the central fibrous body. The node, with its covering of transitional cells, is half oval in shape and sits atop the atrial aspect of the central fibrous body. Because of its shape and location the superior part has potential communication, via the continuation of the central fibrous body and the atrial septum, with both left and right atria. The compact node therefore is an interatrial rather than a purely right atrial structure (Figure 6.4). Because the covering of transitional cells also permits potential communication with both ventricles in the region of the crux cordis, accessory connections can also occur.

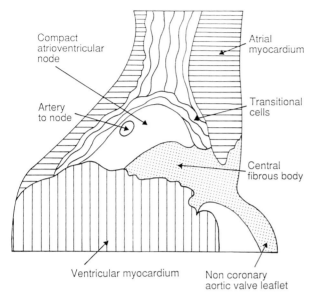

Figure 6.4 Diagram of the atrioventricular junction and the compact atrioventricular node (node of His–Tawara). The compact node is an interatrial rather than a right atrial structure. It is covered with transitional cells which sweep down to make potential connection with ventricular myocardium in both ventricles (see text). The node itself is insulated from the ventricular myocardium by the central fibrous body, through which the common bundle passes before dividing into left and right branches

The connections in this area are commonly recognized by eponyms. Not all of those listed have been identified anatomically.

- Paladino fibres or tracts: accessory septal atrioventricular connection; also transitional nodoventricular bundle.
- Mahaim fibres or tracts: compact nodoventricular bundle; fasciculoventricular connections.
- Atrio-His (sometimes atrioHisian) fibres or tracts: atriofascicular bypass tracts.
- James fibres: intranodal bypass tracts.

Examination of the heart

These are low-risk operations so that early death is unlikely to be attributable to the definitive part of the procedure.

As indicated in Chapter 5, many arrythmogenic foci are epicardial. Unless the ablation was part of an operation needing cardiopulmonary bypass, there is little on the heart to indicate what had been done. After ablation, irrespective of the technique used, the foci appear as small scars. They are not easy to see unless the site was marked (with a stitch, for example) at operation.

The cryoprobe can be applied directly over a coronary artery without risk of perforation[13].

Endocardial ablations

Because interoperative electrophysiological studies are time consuming and expensive, some surgeons prefer to incise the endocardial atrioventricular junction and then suture it. If this has been done, there is no chance of finding the accessory connection, and there are the complications of the procedure itself:

1. Damage to either the great cardiac vein or the circumflex coronary artery, which is deep to the vein and therefore closer to the endocardium. (This of course applies only to left-sided connections. On the right side the right coronary artery is at risk, but it has no concomitant vein).
2. The suture line heals to a raised scar, which in late deaths appears as a supra-annular ring of fibrous tissue and which may cause a degree of mitral stenosis.

If cautery or cryoablation were used the sites are almost impossible to find once they have healed.

References

1. Pritchard, R. W. Tumors of the heart. *Archives of Pathology*, **51**, 98–128, 1951
2. Silverman, N. A. Primary cardiac tumors. *Annals of Surgery*, **191**, 127–138, 1980
3. Larrieu, A. J., Jamieson, W. R. E., Tyers, G. F. O. *et al*. Primary cardiac tumors. *Journal of Thoracic and Cardiovascular Surgery*, **83**, 339–348, 1982
4. Sanodos, G. and Reed, G. E. Primary cardiac sarcomas. *Journal of Thoracic and Cardiovascular Surgery*, **63**, 482–485, 1972
5. Gerbode, F., Kerth, W. J. and Hill, J. D. Surgical management of tumors of the heart. *American Journal of Medicine*, **52**, 9–18, 1972
6. Wenink, A. C. G. Development of the human cardiac conducting system. *Journal of Anatomy*, **121**, 617–631, 1976
7. Anderson, R. H. and Becker, A. E. Anatomy of conducting tissues revisited. *British Heart Journal*, **40** (Supplement), 2–16, 1978
8. Kent, A. F. S. Researches on the structure and function of the mammalian heart. *Journal of Physiology*, **14**, 233–254, 1893
9. Kent, A. F. S. Observations on the auriculo-ventricular junction of the mammalian heart. *Quarterly Journal of Experimental Physiology*, **7**, 193–195, 1913
10. Sealy, W. C., Gallagher, J. J. and Wallace, A. G. The surgical treatment of Wolff–Parkinson–White syndrome. Evolution of improved methods of identification and interruption of the Kent bundle. *Annals of Thoracic Surgery*, **22**, 443–457, 1976
11. Sealy, W. C., Gallagher, J. J. and Pritchett, E. L. C. The surgical anatomy of Kent bundles based on electrophysiological mapping and surgical exploration. *Journal of Thoracic and Cardiovascular Surgery*, **76**, 804–815, 1978
12. Wood, F. C., Wolferth, C. C. and Geckeler, G. D. Histologic demonstration of accessory muscular connections between auricle and ventricle in a case of short P–R interval and prolonged QRS complex. *American Heart Journal*, **25**, 454–462, 1943
13. Misaki, T., Allwork, S. P. and Bentall, H. H. The longterm effects of cryosurgery in the sheep heart. *Cardiovascular Research*, **17**, 61–69, 1983

Part II

Congenital malformations

7

Interatrial communications

Anatomy of the atrial septum
Atrial septal defects
Other interatrial communications

Operations for congenital malformations either modify the anatomy to such an extent that it may be difficult to identify the original morphology, or they remove the anomaly altogether so that it is impossible to recognize at necropsy. These two extremes are well exemplified by transposition of the aorta and pulmonary artery in the first instance, and anomalous pulmonary venous connection in the second. Between the two is a spectrum of findings which holds great potential interest for the prosector.

The first congenital malformation to be corrected with the aid of cardiopulmonary bypass was interatrial communication. Nowadays when it occurs as an isolated anomaly it is almost completely non-fatal, the possible exceptions being mature adult patients (who, in the UK, are almost invariably from abroad), who have severe pulmonary hypertension. Late death may result from uncontrolled anticoagulation because adult patients needing large patches are sometimes anticoagulated for a few months after operation.

While all defects of the atrial septum are interatrial communications, by no means are all interatrial communications atrial septal defects (ASDs)[1].

Anatomy of the atrial septum

The atrial septum is the small area comprising the fossa ovalis and part of the limbus fossa ovalis. The inferior limb of the limbus fossa ovalis is the remnant of the embryonic septum primum and the translucent fossa ovalis is the septum secundum from the embryonic heart. In approximately one-quarter of normal individuals the fossa is incompletely sealed to the limbus so that a small, valvular communication, a 'probe-patent foramen ovale', results.

Atrial septal defects

The ancient habit of naming ASDs according to their speculative embryological origin has caused much confusion in the classification of the anomaly. Traditionally, ASDs were divided into two groups, the so-called 'ostium secundum ASD' and 'ostium primum ASD'. The latter is not a defect of the atrial septum, but of the atrioventricular septum (Chapter 8).

ASDs, by definition, affect the atrial septum. They may be small and with obvious remnants of the fossa ovalis, in which case they are usually quite arbitrarily called 'patent foramen ovale', or they may be so big that the fossa ovalis cannot be identified, in which case they are usually described as 'common atrium'. Most ASDs are between these extremes with respect to size, and they are always related to the atrial septum. Anomalies of pulmonary venous connection are uncommon in these 'genuine' ASDs.

Other interatrial communications

Overriding superior vena cava

In this anomaly the superior vena cava is incompletely incorporated into the right atrium so that it overrides the posterior atrial wall partially to debouch into the left atrium. It is very often associated with anomalies of pulmonary venous connection. Either all the veins from the right lung join the superior vena cava at or close to the cavoatrial junction (hemianomalous pulmonary venous connection), or just one or two veins are thus connected (partially anomalous pulmonary venous connection).

Irrespective of pulmonary venous connections, this anomaly is usually (inappropriately) called 'sinus venosus defect' or, worse, 'sinus venosus ASD', despite the fact that the atrial septum is not involved in the anomaly.

Less commonly, the inferior vena cava overrides and may carry one (usually that from the lower lobe) or more pulmonary veins.

Coronary sinus

The fate of the left horn of the embryonic sinus venosus is to become the coronary sinus, but the vein persists in a number of normal individuals as a 'left superior vena cava' which opens (as a normal connection) into the coronary sinus, which may be greatly enlarged (aneurysmal coronary sinus). As with the right superior vena cava, the left superior vena cava sometimes carries either or both the pulmonary veins, thus becoming anomalous.

Sinus septum defects

The wall between the great cardiac vein (or left superior vena cava 'replacing' it) and the left atrium is called the sinus septum. If the vein fails to reach the right atrium, opening instead beneath the posterior wall of the atrium, it straddles in a manner similar to that of an overriding vena cava; such a defect is called an unroofed coronary sinus.

If the sinus septum is deficient in the left atrium, the resulting defect is called a sinus septum defect.

To summarize the anatomy of interatrial communications:

1. ASDs:
   (a) Are always related to the fossa ovalis.
   (b) May be large.
   (c) Are seldom associated with anomalies of either pulmonary or systemic venous connection (unless anomalies of visceral situs are present).
   (d) Are very often associated with complex congenital cardiac malformations.
2. Other interatrial communications:
   (a) Are not related to the fossa ovalis.
   (b) Are usually small.
   (c) Are frequently associated with anomalies of both pulmonary and systemic venous connection.
   (d) Are often associated with complex congenital cardiac malformations and also with ASDs.

Operations for ASD generally utilize a patch to close the defect, which is often large, but persistent foramen ovale is usually closed by direct suture. Operations for other interatrial communications also necessitate the use of a patch, and as the procedure re-routes venous return to its appropriate atrium the patch may need to be quite large.

As previously stated, death following operation in isolated interatrial communication is almost unknown today, while, in complex malformations, that part of the repair is seldom implicated. However, there are a few complications:

1. Disruption of the patch, due perhaps to a section of continuous suture giving

way, or to interrupted sutures cutting out of a too small patch. Sepsis is a rare cause of patch disruption.

2. 'Tenting-up' of either atrium or veins, with consequent obstruction, of too small a re-routing patch.
3. Kinking, also causing obstruction, of too large a re-routing patch.
4. In late death of patients operated on in babyhood, outgrowth of the repair, with consequent obstruction to either systemic or pulmonary venous drainage.
5. Fatal bleeding, e.g. into the gut, due to escape from anticoagulant control.

Reference

1. Allwork, S. P. Anatomical versus embryological nomenclature in cardiac malformations exemplified by interatrial communications. *Theoretical Surgery*, **2**, 129–132, 1987

8

Atrioventricular septal defect

Atrioventricular septal defect (AVSD) is a complex and surgically challenging malformation which has been recognized, like most congenital cardiac malformations, for at least 150 years, but its true nature, i.e. that it is not an anomaly of atrial septation, has been appreciated only relatively recently.

A discussion of the history of the nomenclature and classification of AVSD is beyond the scope of this book, but is to be found elsewhere[1–4]. A short description of the morphology with some reference to the developmental anatomy of the heart is given to clarify this complex anomaly.

Anatomy

The atrioventricular muscular septum is a small triangular wedge of muscle which interposes between the left ventricle and the right atrium. It lies posteroinferior to the membranous part of the ventricular septum, from which it is distinct. Both the atrioventricular valves are attached to it, the tricuspid slightly more apically than the mitral[1,5] (Figure 8.1). This structure is confluent with the posterior, inlet part of the ventricular septum from which the atrioventricular valves developed in the embryonic heart[6].

The inlet septum separates the ventricular inlets and wedges the aortic valve between them. The inlet septum is roughly triangular and its surface is smooth. It accounts for approximately one-third of the septal mass and is recognized in the right ventricle as the septal muscle extending from the posterior wall of the heart to the trabecula septomarginalis (which is called the 'moderator band' in some US literature). The posterior (inferior) and infundibular (septal) papillary muscles of the tricuspid valve arise from the inlet septum. (In the right ventricle there is no tensor apparatus anterior to the trabecula septomarginalis, which marks the boundary between inlet and outlet septa) (Figure 8.2a). In the left ventricle the inlet septum is recognized as the smooth triangle of muscular septum extending from the interventricular membranous septum (just beneath the left leaflet of the aortic valve) posteriorly, under the mitral valve, towards the crux cordis (Figure 8.2b).

From the foregoing it is evident that absence of the atrioventricular muscular septum will result in a gap between the lower edge of the atrial septum and the upper border of the ventricular septum, and that, as the atrioventricular valves should have been attached to the missing septum, they too might demonstrate some abnormalities (Figure 8.3).

AVSD is characterized by:

1. A defect between the lower rim of the atrial septum and the upper margin of the ventricular septum.
2. A degree of derangement of the atrioventricular valves, particularly the left one.
3. ASD *may* coexist, but often the atrial septum is intact.

In AVSD the absence of the atrioventricular septum is usually associated with a degree of deficiency of the inlet septum, with which it is confluent, so that a spectrum of anomalies is expressed. It is the breadth of this spectrum and the diversity of morphological characteristics within it which has traditionally made the anomaly so difficult to classify. The major difficulties concern the status of the atrioventricular valves and the presence or absence of a septal deficiency below the atrioventricular valves.

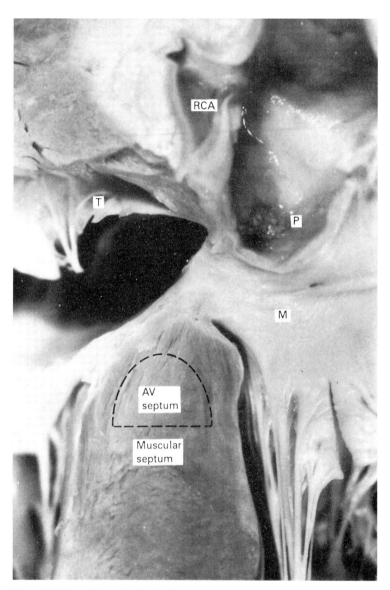

Figure 8.1 The atrioventricular (AV) muscular septum separates the left and right inflow tracts. Both the mitral (M) and tricuspid (T) leaflets are attached to it, the tricuspid rather more apically than the mitral. The aortic valve leaflets have been removed. RCA, ostium of the right coronary artery; P, posterior (non-coronary) aortic sinus. (From *Thoracic and Cardiovascular Surgeon*, by permission)

Atrioventricular valves

Because there is almost always a degree of inlet septum deficit, there is almost always a degree of derangement of the atrioventricular valves. As these valves have been developed abnormally, due to the inlet septum malformation, they have lost their normal morphology, i.e. a major anterior leaflet and a longer but shallower

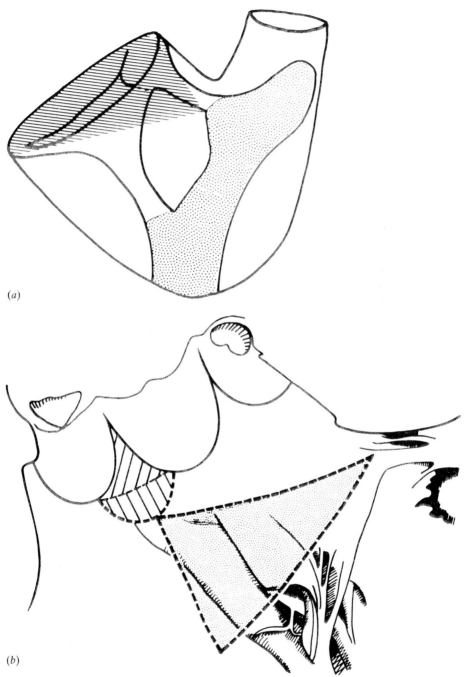

(a)

(b)

Figure 8.2 (a) Diagram of the right ventricle to indicate the extent of the inlet septum (hatched). The trabecula septomarginalis (stippled) marks the anterior boundary of the inlet septum, and the tricuspid tensor apparatus does not extend anterior to this structure. (b) Diagram of the inlet septum (stippled) seen from the left ventricle. It is inferior and posterior to the membranous part of the ventricular septum (hatched). The inlet musculature gives anteroposterior depth to the basal part of the left ventricle

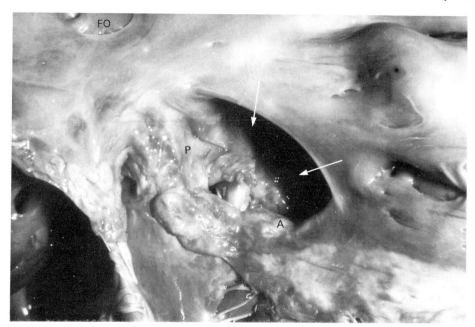

Figure 8.3 Atrioventricular septal defect (arrowed), with intact atrial septum and incompletely partitioned, abnormal atrioventricular valves (Rastelli type A). FO, fossa ovalis; A, anterior leaflet of the common valve; P, posterior leaflet of the common valve

scalloped leaflet on the left, the whole looking somewhat like a bishop's mitre, and a well defined anterior leaflet and medial and posterior leaflets with papillary muscles all either arising from the septum or very close to it on the right. Instead, the atrioventricular valves demonstrate a great diversity of morphology, but there are some constant characteristics.

Left atrioventricular valve

In AVSD the left atrioventricular valve loses its bileaflet structure and therefore ceases to be a 'mitral' valve. Instead, it has three leaflets: anterior, posterior (or septal) and lateral (Figure 8.4a). The papillary muscles are often poorly developed, and appear to be placed rather high up, due to the absence of inlet septum muscle. Similarly, the valve leaflets are often poorly developed and may be either dysplastic or verrucous. The disposition of the anterior leaflet is variable and the valve may be partially attached to the left ventricular outflow tract, narrowing it[7].

The 'cleft'

In almost all hearts with AVSD there is a gap between the anterior and posterior leaflets of the left atrioventricular valve which exposes the summit of the ventricular septum (Figure 8.4a). This gap is usually (perhaps confusingly) called a 'cleft anterior leaflet', although the anterior leaflet is never cloven in two. Instead, absence of the atrioventricular septum, to which the leaflets are normally attached, permits a commissure between the anterior and posterior leaflets. This abnormal commissure may be relatively large, but even when small, the absence of tensor

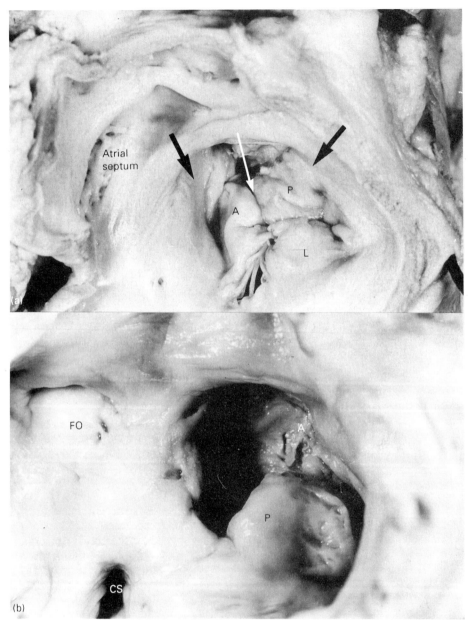

Figure 8.4 (a) The left atrioventricular valve in AVSD. There are three leaflets (A, anterior; P, posterior; L, lateral) so that the valve has lost its mitral morphology. The space (small arrow) between the anterior and posterior leaflets is the so-called cleft anterior leaflet. The leaflet itself is never cloven, the space between the leaflets is a commissure, unsupported by subvalvular tensor apparatus. The 'cleft' permits left ventricle to right atrium shunting in a proportion of cases. The AVSD itself (large arrows) is beneath the intact atrial septum. (b) The right atrioventricular valve in AVSD in the same heart. The posterior leaflet (P) is dysplastic and bridges the muscular septum. The usupported commissure (the 'cleft') is between the anterior (A) and posterior bridging leaflets. CS, coronary sinus; FO, fossa ovalis. (From *British Heart Journal*, by permission)

apparatus may make it regurgitant. Thus there is a potential for shunting from left ventricle to right atrium.

Accessory orifices

Accessory orifices, developmentally and morphologically identical to the so-called cleft, occur with some frequency between the posterior and lateral leaflets, and also between the anterior and lateral leaflets. They are relatively unimportant as they do not leak to cause regurgitation, but as they are sometimes quite large their appearance may seem ominous.

Right atrioventricular valve

Like the left valve, the right has anterior, posterior and lateral leaflets (Figure 8.4b). Similarly, they are abnormally arranged and may be dysplastic.

Common atrioventricular valve

When the atrioventricular valve is incompletely separated into two, or where there is no separation at all, the valve is called a common valve. This anomaly is seen in other congenital cardiac malformations as well, but is a fairly common finding in AVSD. The morphology of this common valve is variable with respect to the disposition of the two major leaflets, but anterior and posterior leaflets are recognized, together with left and right lateral leaflets[3,4].

Outflow tracts

The *left* ventricular outflow tract is attenuated in this malformation due to absence of the muscular atrioventricular septum and the inlet septum deficiency. The inlet septum gives the normal left ventricular outflow tract its anteroposterior dimension and this is lost when the inlet septum is absent or deficient. Furthermore, the aortic valve is wedged between the ventricular inlets in the normal heart by the atrioventricular septum, and this wedged position is also lost when the septum is absent, so that the aortic valve is a little superior and to the right of its normal position.

When there is a large septal defect the left atrioventricular valve may attach to the edge of the outlet septum so that it narrows the left ventricular outflow, as well as being abnormal in itself. It is this combination of morphology which gives the characteristic appearance at left ventricular angiography of the fancifully-named 'goose-neck', so beloved by paediatric cardiologists.

Narrowing of the left ventricular outlet may be aggravated by hypertrophy of the outlet septum, expressed as a bulging infundibular septum beneath the right aortic valve leaflet. (The morphology of this muscle bears no resemblance whatever to the discrete bulge sometimes seen in hypertrophic cardiomyopathy (idiopathic hypertrophic subaortic stenosis). There is no danger of confusing them!)

The *right* outflow may show a number of anomalies, such as infundibular and/or valvular stenosis, hypoplasia or atresia. Anomalies of ventriculoarterial connection, such as double outlet right ventricle or arterial transposition, occur in patients with trisomies, particularly trisomy 21, but are not confined to them.

Classification

From the foregoing paragraphs it is evident that there is a wide range of malformations within the compass of AVSD, and these have been variously classified during the last 100 years. Although this gives a fine potential for confusion, classification of AVSD is capable of clarification.

Rokitansky was the first to offer a classification in 1875[8]. He divided the hearts into three groups, and, as was his almost invariable practice, he considered the embryological derivation in each case; he then named the groups accordingly. Rokitansky termed the whole group 'atrioventricular canal defects' and the name has, unfortunately, persisted to the present day. The first of Rokitansky's subgroups held those hearts in which only the atrioventricular septum was absent; there was no defect below the completely separated atrioventricular valves. These were designated 'ostium primum ASD', as Rokitansky did not recognize the atrioventricular septum, considering instead that a defect above the atrioventricular valves concerned the atrial septum, while one beneath them was a defect of the ventricular septum. When the defect was coupled with a deficit of left atrioventricular valve tissue so that there was a gap (the cleft) on the summit of the ventricular septum, the defect was designated a 'partial atrioventricular canal'. If these anomalies were accompanied by a septal defect beneath the atrioventricular valves he called the anomaly a 'complete atrioventricular canal'. The distinction between the partial (i.e. without a VSD) and complete (with a VSD) forms of the malformation has lasted to the present day, and is still widely employed.

In 1948, Rogers and Edwards[9] restudied the malformation and followed the established nomenclature.

In 1956, Wakai and Edwards[10] returned to AVSD, with particular attention to the atrioventricular valves. In that extensive study the partial form had two completely separated atrioventricular valves (with or without cleft), and without a ventricular septal defect. The complete form had a common atrioventricular valve and a VSD. They also noted a third kind, which they designated a 'transitional' sort, in which the valves were almost completely separated, as a tongue of valve tissue almost covered the summit of the septum. However, of the hearts in that group, several also had a VSD, so that a potential for confusion was introduced.

At the beginning of the surgical era for congenital heart disease, Watkins and Gross in the USA called the defect an 'endocardial cushion defect'[11] and at approximately the same time, Bedford et al. in England introduced the term 'atrioventricular defect'[12]. The current name (atrioventricular septal defect) had been used in speech for several years before its first appearance in print as a title in 1982[1].

In 1979, Piccoli et al. described a large series of hearts, also naming them atrioventricular defects, and classified them as partial or complete defects according to whether the atrioventricular valves were separate (partial) or not (complete)[3,4].

Thus there are two criteria for partial and complete defects. The first uses septal defect below the atrioventricular valve(s) to identify complete defect, while the second, newer definition, uses the status of the atrioventricular valves.

Rastelli's classification[13,14] (Figure 8.5) was the first to address the problems of the atrioventricular valves from a purely surgical standpoint. The designations concerned only the complete form, with interventricular communication. In type A, the atrioventricular valves were almost separate, with chordal attachments to

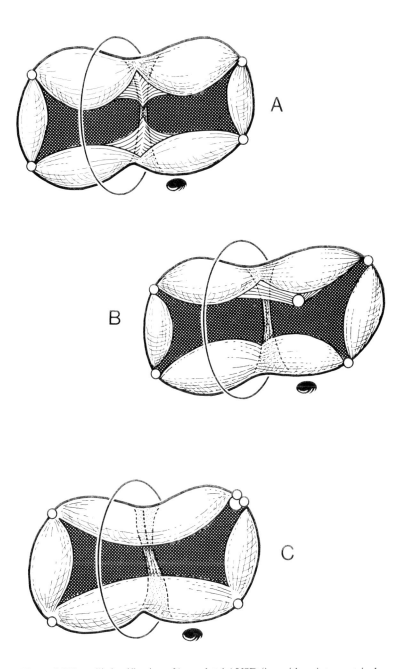

Figure 8.5 Rastelli classification of 'complete' AVSD (i.e. with an interventricular communication beneath the common atrioventricular valve seen from above). Type A has two almost separated valves whose anterior and posterior leaflets bridge the muscular septum. Both leaflets are attached to this slightly concave septal summit. Type B has the anterior leaflet bridging the septum, and as tensor apparatus from its left component passes to the right ventricle the left component straddles the septum. Type C has both anterior and posterior leaflets bridging the septum, but without straddling

the ventricular septum. Type B had the left anterior leaflet straddling the ventricular septum, with a papillary muscle in the right ventricle, while the posterior leaflet was more or less attached to the septum and with evenly distributed tensor apparatus. In type C, both anterior and posterior leaflets bridged the septum (bridging leaflets). The papillary muscles supported only the lateral commissures of the valve.

Surgical treatment of the malformation is concerned primarily with remodelling the atrioventricular valve(s). The septal defect, even though it may be of spectacular size, is not usually problematical to the surgeon. Thus, in the surgical era, the classifications based on atrioventricular valve morphology are more useful when planning operations than are the older ones.

The operation

Of all complex congenital malformations of the heart, AVSD, by its infinite variety, probably presents the surgeon with as great a challenge as is likely to be encountered in the surgery of congenital heart disease. No other anomaly demands such attention to every detail of the anatomy in each individual, nor such ingenuity on the part of the surgeon to make the most of the often poorly developed tissues.

The valves

As the majority of patients with this disorder are children, or even babies, the atrioventricular valves are not replaced with prostheses unless absolutely unavoidable, e.g. grossly inadequate or unusable leaflet tissue, or (rare) infection. In most patients only the left valve or left component of a common valve needs radical remodelling. In the case of a common valve it has also to be appropriately apportioned to the two ventricles and this depends to a considerable extent upon the placement of the patch used to close the septal defect. Success depends upon the achievement of two competent valves. This is mandatory in the case of the left one as the left atrium is often small in these hearts, and regurgitation is intolerable to it. Refashioning of the valve is done by incising the leaflets where necessary and attaching them to the patch appropriately. It is sometimes possible to split the papillary muscles to provide a bigger orifice, and also to 'unroll' thick, verrucous leaflets to enlarge the leaflet size.

The 'cleft'

Although it is almost always present, the cleft is regurgitant in only about a third of cases. In those cases where it is regurgitant, successful management depends upon making the valve competent without making it stenotic. Mild stenosis is far better tolerated than even an apparently trivial degree of regurgitation. When the cleft is sutured, the knots are tied, sometimes over a pledget on the ventricular aspect. It is unusual to close the whole length from the annulus to the free edges.

The patch

Depending on the size of the defect, either one or two patches are used. When there is a defect below the atrioventricular valve(s) a single patch often suffices, but when elaborate refashioning of the valves is needed, separate patches above and below the valves may be more appropriate. Either pericardium (autologous or heterologous), or knitted Dacron or felt may be used. Felt is less commonly used today because lighter and more supple materials are available; it is more or less confined to subvalvular use and to pledgets.

Associated anomalies

Concomitant right ventricular outflow tract obstruction (see Chapter 12) adds to the risk of operation, and its relief may necessitate the use of more prosthetic material. Palliative operations such as a Blalock or Waterston procedure (see Chapter 11) are taken down at the time of radical operation.

Obstruction to the left ventricular outflow tract may be treated at the same operation, but as it tends to develop slowly in the months following the radical operation, this is rare.

The ductus arteriosus is usually closed in a separate, earlier procedure, but if it is small, or was palliating pulmonary stenosis, it may be left until the radical operation. It is closed either by ligation with ductus tape (round and braided) or with umbilical tape (flat and braided). Metal clips, such as brain clips, are also used for this purpose. The duct can also be divided between ligatures or clips.

Coarctation of the aorta, like ductus arteriosus, is usually treated in a separate, earlier operation, and the duct, if present, is tied then.

Pulmonary artery band

The purpose of this procedure is to reduce the pulmonary blood flow. It is now largely obsolete as more patients are treated at ever younger ages. The band, usually of tape, as above, is tied or sutured into place as a closed procedure in infancy. At the definitive operation it is removed. This removal is made difficult when the band has been in place for some time as it causes a vigorous reaction, eventually working its way into the lumen of the pulmonary artery. It must then be treated by excision and application of a patch graft to the pulmonary artery.

Examination of the heart

AVSD exemplifies to a marked degree the advantages of examination of the fixed heart over that of the fresh specimen. Assessment of the status of the repaired valves is virtually impossible if their morphology is lost due to cutting through the annuli in an unfixed specimen. If it is considered necessary, small transverse incisions may be made in the atria to assist the removal of blood for better fixation, but as the right atrium is almost invariably markedly enlarged, it should seldom be necessary.

The valves

After evaluation of the suture lines and incisions for cardiopulmonary bypass (see Chapter 1), incise the right atrium from the appendage to the inferior vena cava to show the atrial septum, the patched atrioventricular septum and the right atrioventricular valve. Competence of the valve may be tested by putting the specimen in water, although it is always rather less informative for the right atrioventricular valve than for the left, irrespective of the diagnosis. In the case of a common valve the anterior bridging leaflet will have been divided anteriorly and stitched to the patch. The posterior leaflet may have been similarly treated. Check the suture lines, as occasionally a stitch may cut out if there was a big tissue deficit.

Open the left atrium from the right upper lobe pulmonary vein to the atrial appendage to display the left side of the patch and the remodelled left atrioventricular valve. (If a prosthesis was used it is best seen and examined by this approach.) The remodelled valve will have either two or three leaflets, depending upon what tissue was available. The new leaflets are disposed so that there is a major anteromedial one, usually with a suture line from the annulus to a variable distance from the free edge, a smaller posteromedial one, and the unchanged lateral leaflet. After assessing the competence of the valve and the suture lines, as for the right side, the annulus may be cut to see the left ventricle. As the specimen is fixed, the morphology of the valve is retained and can be demonstrated at any time.

The ventricles and the patch(es)

The right ventricle may be opened by an incision extending from the atrial side of the acute margin of the heart to the apex of the right ventricle, then upwards through the pulmonary outflow tract, having due regard to any modification of the outflow tract.

If there was an interventricular component to the defect the patch is visible under the new right atrioventricular valve, which will form the roof of the repair. If two patches were used there will be a suture line under the valve; if there is one patch, part of the right atrioventricular valve will be sewn to it.

If there is an outflow tract patch the underlying structures are best seen if, after examining the suture lines, a small opening is made with scissors in the middle of the patch. The small cut can then be extended vertically in each direction, under direct vision, to preserve the subjacent anatomy.

The left ventricle is opened through the obtuse margin to the apex, then upwards to the aortic outflow tract. The left ventricle demonstrates the pathognomonic discrepancy between the length of the inlet and outlet portions of the chamber. As the inlet septum accounts for about a third of the septal mass, up to a third of it may be missing in AVSD, so that instead of the inlet and outlet measurements being, for practical purposes, the same, the inlet may be only a third of the outlet[1,3,4]. The remainder (the defect) is occupied by the patch to which the new left anterioventricular valve is likely to be attached (i.e. if there had been a common valve with a bridging leaflet, or if the anterior leaflet had been (abnormally) attached to the outlet septum[1,10]. The leaflet will now either be divided (bridging leaflet) or be detached from the left ventricular outflow tract and resutured to the patch. As on the right side, the valve forms the roof of the repair in most cases.

Anticipated findings

Early death

1. Complications of cardiopulmonary bypass (see Chapter 1).
2. Pulmonary oedema resulting from acute pulmonary hypertension due to left atrioventricular valve regurgitation.

3. Pulmonary oedema resulting from acute pulmonary hypertension due to iatrogenic left atrioventricular valve stenosis.
4. Disruption of a part of the repair, due perhaps to dysplastic valve tissue or a slightly too small patch.
5. Haemorrhage or oedema around the common atrioventricular bundle. (The bundle is abnormally long in AVSD as its normally short route to the membranous septum, where it bifurcates, is, of course, absent.)
6. Pre-existing pulmonary hypertension.

Late death

1. Cardiomegaly.
2. Fibrosis of the common dundle. Arrythmias are common in AVSD as life advances, and are part of the natural history of the malformation.
3. Disruption of part of the repair.
   (a) In patients with dysplastic valves the tissue may tear, particularly at the annulus, close to the repair of the cleft (Figure 8.6).

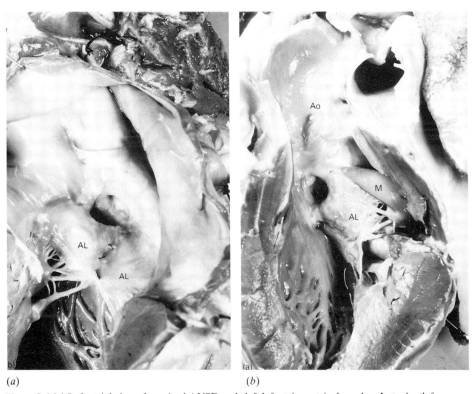

(a)   (b)

Figure 8.6 (a) Left atrial view of repaired AVSD and cleft left atrioventricular valve. Late death from arrythmia in an adult patient. The sutures apposing the edges of the cleft are visible on the atrial aspect of the anterior leaflet (AL) which has contracted away from the healed patch, permitting a left ventricle–left atrium communication. (b) Ventricular view. The site of the tear corresponds to the area of aortomitral continuity in the normal heart. The chordae tendineae of the atrioventricular valve are short and poorly developed and part of the anterior papillary muscle group (M) inserts directly into the leaflet. Ao, aorta. (Reproduced by permission of Springer-Verlag)

(b) Very rarely the defect may reopen in patients operated upon long ago (e.g. adults treated in childhood). If an incomplete diagnosis was made then, they were sometimes treated as ASDs and small defects were closed by direct suture, which eventually gives way.

4. Acquired left atrioventricular valve stenosis associated with closure of the cleft.
5. Acquired aortic outflow tract obstruction. The infundibular septum can hypertrophy after operation and obstruct the left ventricular outflow.
6. Right atrioventricular valve regurgitation and/or stenosis.
7. Pulmonary hypertension.
8. Infective endocarditis.
9. Problems associated with prosthetic heart valves, where used (see Chapter 3).

References

1. Allwork, S. P. Anatomical embryological correlates in atrioventricular septal defect. *British Heart Journal*, **47**, 419–429, 1982
2. Wenink, A. C. G. Embryology of the ventricular septum. *Virchows Archiv; Abteilung A: Pathologische Anatomie*, **390**, 71–79, 1981
3. Piccoli, G. P., Gerlis, L. M., Wilkinson, J. L. *et al.* Morphology and classification of atrioventricular defects. *British Heart Journal*, **42**, 621–632, 1979
4. Piccoli, G. P., Wilkinson, J. L., Gerlis, L. M. and Anderson, R. H. Morphology and classification of complete atrioventricular defects. *British Heart Journal*, **42**, 633–639, 1979
5. Allwork, S. P. The anatomical basis of infection of the aortic root. *Thoracic and Cardiovascular Surgeon*, **34**, 143–148, 1986
6. Wenink, A. C. G. and Gittenberger de Groot, A. C. The role of atrioventricular cushions in the septation of the heart. *International Journal of Cardiology*, **8**, 25–44, 1985
7. Allwork, S. P. The mitral valve in complete atrioventricular canal defect. In *Cardiovascular Surgery 1980* (eds W. Bircks, J. Ostermeyer and H. D. Schulte), Springer-Verlag, Berlin, pp. 357–361, 1981
8. Rokitansky, C. *Die Defekte der Scheidewande des Herzens. Pathologisch-anatomisch Abhandlung.* Braumuller, Vienna, 1875
9. Rogers, H. M. and Edwards, J. E. Incomplete division of the atrioventricular canal with patent interatrial foramen primum (persistent common atrioventricular ostium). *American Heart Journal*, **36**, 28–54, 1948
10. Wakai, C. S. and Edwards, J. E. Developmental and pathologic considerations in persistent common atrioventricular canal. *Proceedings of the Staff Meetings of the Mayo Clinic*, **31**, 487–500, 1956
11. Watkins, E. and Gross, R. E. Experience with surgical repair of atrial septal defect. *Journal of Thoracic Surgery*, **30**, 469–491, 1955
12. Bedford, D. E., Sellors, T. H., Somerville, W. *et al.* Atrial septal defect and its surgical treatment. *Lancet*, **ii**, 1255–1261, 1957
13. Rastelli, G., Kirklin, J. W. and Titus, J. Anatomic observation on complete form of persistent common atrioventricular canal with special reference to the atrioventricular valves. *Mayo Clinic Proceedings*, **41**, 296–308, 1966
14. Rastelli, G., Ongley, P. A., Kirklin, J. W. and McGoon, G. C. Surgical repair of the complete form of common atrioventricular canal. *Journal of Thoracic and Cardiovascular Surgery*, **55**, 299–308, 1968

9

Anomalies of pulmonary venous connection

This anomaly was first described by Wilson in 1798[1], but the condition was not treatable surgically until the 1950s[2]. The more common 'partial' and 'hemianomalous' connections are considered in Chapter 7, together with interatrial communications.

The malformation is rare as an isolated anomaly, but is part of the disorder in asplenia and polysplenia syndromes.

Totally anomalous pulmonary venous connection (TAPVC) is classified according to the site of the anomalous connection. In descending order of frequency[3], these are:

- Supracardiac: to the left innominate vein $\left.\begin{array}{l} \\ \end{array}\right\}$ >50%
                  to the right superior vena cava
                  to a left superior vena cava
                  to the azygos vein.
- Intracardiac: to the coronary sinus
                  to the right atrium.
- Infracardiac: to the inferior vena cava *or*
                  to a persistent ductus venosus.
- Mixed: to a combination of the above, and (rarely) to other abdominal
                  veins.

Supracardiac TAPVC is often accompanied by heart failure in life; obstruction is very rare. By contrast, in intracardiac TAPVC obstruction is relatively common. The pulmonary veins are obstructed, either at the confluence or within the parenchyma of the lungs, so that pulmonary vascular obstructive disease is present.

Interatrial communication, usually a widely patent foramen ovale, is always present and there is nearly always a ductus arteriosus.

Hypoplasia of the left atrium and left ventricle are sometimes associated with TAPVC, but other intracardiac malformations are rare.

The operation

Supracardiac   The vertical vein is ligated and the horizontal confluence of the pulmonary veins is incised lengthwise and anastomosed to a corresponding incision in the left atrium. Some or all of this anastomosis is done with interrupted sutures to allow for the baby's subsequent growth. The interatrial communication is usually closed through a separate right atriotomy using a patch.

Intracardiac   The coronary sinus is fenestrated into the left atrium and its original opening closed, usually by oversewing. The ASD is patched.

Infracardiac   In contrast to the supracardiac type, in infracardiac TAPVC the confluence of the veins is most often a vertical vessel and the widest anastomosis is gained by low division of this vein and as large a vertical incision in the left atrium as is practicable.

As there is almost always a ductus arteriosus, this is ligated, or, less commonly, divided.

Necropsy

Early death

Despite great reductions in surgical mortality in recent years, it remains high in TAPVC. Because the condition often requires surgical operation so early in life, death in the immediate postoperative period is usually due to factors other than those resulting directly from the operation, for example, the patient's pre-existing metabolic state. Complications of cardiopulmonary bypass (see Chapter 1) may be implicated in these patients. Of factors directly related to the operation, failure radically to improve the haemodynamic status because of hypoplasia of the left atrium and/or ventricle may be contributory.

It is sometimes very hard to find the original anomalous vein, especially in infracardiac connections, and may be impossible unless it is sought before removing the thoracic contents from the body.

On no account should the heart and lungs be separated as this renders assessment of the anastomoses impossible. It also precludes injection of the veins, if this is desired.

Suture lines   Occasionally the suture line obstructs a pulmonary vein, or causes kinking. In intracardiac TAPVC there may be a haematoma in the right atrium causing or aggravating arrythmia because of proximity of the coronary sinus to the common bundle.

Late death

Late mortality is nearly always due to persistent pulmonary arterial hypertension consequent upon pulmonary venous hypertension. The cause of this is either recurrent or residual pulmonary venous obstruction. In the latter case it may be the result of the child having outgrown the repair, but pulmonary vascular obstructive disease may also be implicated and endocardial thickening at the anastomotic site may be contributory.

References

1. Wilson, J. A description of a very unusual malformation of the human heart. *Philosophical Transactions of the Royal Society of London*, **88**, 346–356, 1798
2. Norwood, W. I. and Castaneda, A. R. Disorders of pulmonary venous return. In *Davis–Christopher Textbook of Surgery* (ed. D. C. Sabiston), W. B. Saunders, Philadelphia, pp. 2247–2252, 1981
3. Mathew, R., Thilenius, O. G., Replogle, R. L. *et al.* Cardiac function in total anomalous pulmonary venous return before and after surgery. *Circulation*, **55**, 361–370, 1977

10

Defects of the ventricular septum

Isolated ventricular septal defect (VSD) accounts for 30–40% of all congenital cardiac malformations at birth, but up to half of them close spontaneously during the first 3 years of life[1]. VSDs may be grouped into two major categories, according to their anatomical location: perimembranous/malalignment VSD and muscular VSD. These categories may be subdivided according to which *component of* the septum is affected, and for this purpose an outline of the anatomy of the ventricular septum is given. Unlike the interventricular communications due to myocardial infarction (see Chapter 5), congenital VSDs all have well-defined boundaries.

Anatomy

Ventricular septum

The ventricular septum reflects its multifocal origin in its morphology. It has three zones: the *inlet* (described in Chapter 8), the *trabecular* (apical) and the *outlet* (infundibular) zones.

The inlet septum is smooth when examined from either ventricle, and occupies about a third of the septal mass. The trabecular septum is continuous with it, accounting for approximately a fifth of the whole, and lies apically. The outlet septum is the most anterior element and continues from the trabecular apex to the pulmonary valve in the right ventricle. In the left ventricle this outlet septum is represented by the small muscular portion of the left ventricular outflow tract beneath the right aortic sinus (see Chapter 4). This last region, which separates the aortic and pulmonary outflow tracts, is called the *infundibular septum* (Figure 10.1a).

When seen from the right ventricle, there is a translucent area traversing the commissure between the posterior and medial leaflets of the tricuspid valve. This is the membranous part of the ventricular septum (Figure 10.1b). It has two components, an *interventricular* and a *ventriculoatrial* part. When examined from

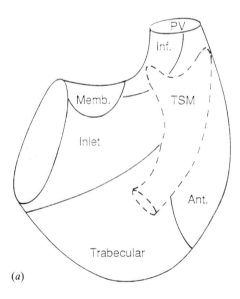

(a)

Figure 10.1 (a) Diagram of the right ventricle to indicate the location of the elements of the ventricular septum. The membranous part of the ventricular septum (Memb.) and infundibular septum (Inf.), together with the ventriculoinfundibular fold (not shown), separate the tricuspid valve from the pulmonary valve (PV). The inlet part occupies about a third of the septal mass. The apical, trabecular portion is confluent with the anterior (Ant.) outlet septum. The trabecula septomarginalis (TSM) marks the boundary between inlet and outlet portions

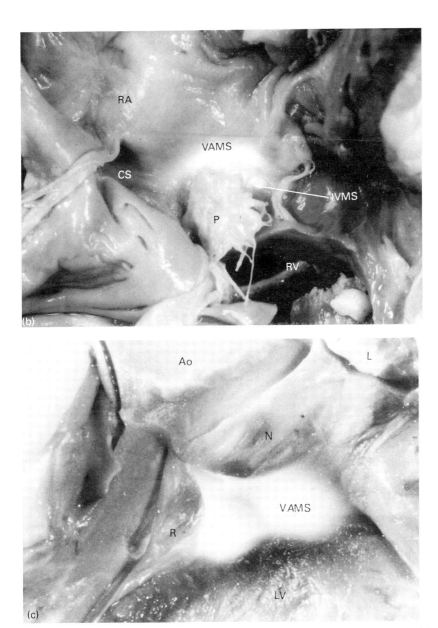

Figure 10.1 continued (b) The membranous part of the ventricular septum seen from the right side of the heart. The ventriculoarterial portion (VAMS), which is large in this elderly individual, lies above the tricuspid valve. The interventricular component (IVMS, arrowed) is smaller. There is a gap between the posterior tricuspid leaflet (P) and the anterior leaflet. Tricuspid valve morphology alters as life advances, and the common finding of a very large membranous septum in old hearts may help to explain not only tricuspid regurgitation in right ventricular volume overload, but sudden onset of arrythmias including complete heart block, in old people. CS, coronary sinus; RA, right atrium; RV, right ventricle. (c) Left ventricular view of the membranous part of the ventricular septum. The small interventricular portion between the right (R) and posterior, non-coronary (N) leaflets of the aortic valve is separated from the ventriculoarterial part (VAMS) by the tricuspid valve (indicated by a wire passed beneath it). Ao, aorta; L, left aortic valve leaflet; LV, left ventricle

the left ventricle, the membranous part lies beneath the aortic valve. It is bounded on the left by the area of aortomitral fibrous continuity and extends from the left aortic sinus to the left-hand edge of the right aortic sinus (Figure 10.1c).

Ventricular septal defects

Perimembranous/malalignment VSDs (Figure 10.2)

These account for approximately three-quarters of all isolated VSDs except among Japanese patients (see below). The defect is usually considerably larger than the membranous septum, and this structure is usually identifiable [2]. Malalignment of the inlet and outlet portions is often plainly visible (Figure 10.2b). The defect has a fibrous posterior boundary, formed by the membranous septum. This permits

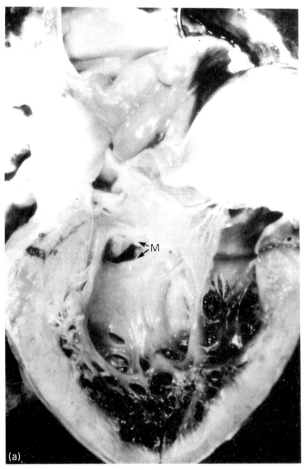

Figure 10.2 (a) Left ventricular view of a perimembranous/malalignment ventricular septal defect (VSD). The defect is beneath the aortic valve, but separated from it by a slip of muscle, due to the malalignment of inlet and outlet septa. The membranous septum (M) forms the posterior border of the defect, through which the tricuspid valve is visible

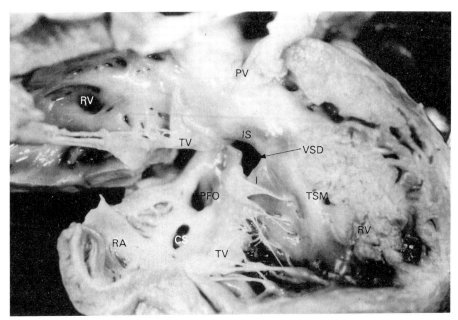

Figure 10.2 continued (b) Right-sided view of the same heart. The VSD lies between the inlet septum (I) and the infundibular septum (IS). CS, coronary sinus; PFO, patent foramen ovale; PV, pulmonary valve; RA, right atrium; RV, right ventricle; TSM, trabecula septomarginalis; TV, tricuspid valve

fibrous continuity between the tricuspid, aortic and mitral valves. The common bundle lies in this fibrous tissue and usually bifurcates there, but it may pass anteriorly for some distance before dividing. The location of the bundle with respect to its depth in the myocardium is variable.

Perimembranous/malalignment VSDs may be large and extend posteriorly into the myocardium inlet septum, anteriorly into the outlet region, or, if the defect is very big indeed, into the trabecular zone. VSDs extending into the outlet septum may reach the pulmonary valve, in which case they are additionally classified as *subarterial* VSDs.

Muscular VSDs (Figure 10.3a)

These occur at the junctional areas of the ventricular septum and may be multiple. Similarly they can be either small or large.

Infundibular muscular VSDs have entirely muscular borders and are remote from the atrioventricular bundle. The defects may either represent malalignment of the anterior and infundibular septa and be located close to the (intact and transilluminable) membranous septum, or they may result from absence of the infundibular septum so that they are subarterial. It is the latter type which predominates among Japanese, but they account for only about a quarter of VSDs in the rest of the world. Absence of the infundibular septum may permit prolapse of

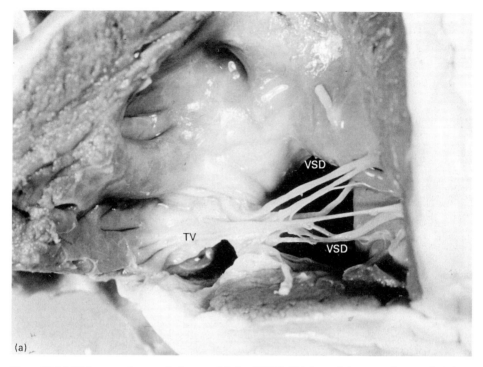

Figure 10.3 (a) Inlet muscular ventricular septal defect (VSD). This large defect extends posteriorly into the inlet septum and is roofed by the (dysplastic) tricuspid valve (TV)

the right, and sometimes the posterior leaflets of the aortic valve through the defect, so that aortic valve regurgitation may be associated.

Infundibular muscular VSDs are sometimes called supracristal or subpulmonary VSDs. The crista supraventricularis is the arch of muscle composed of the ventriculoinfundibular fold, the infundibular septum and the trabecula septomarginalis, which in the normal heart separates the inlet and outlet portions of the right ventricle[3]. However, in congenitally malformed hearts one or more of these elements may be either absent or displaced, so that the term is then inappropriate.

Although the subpulmonary VSD, when seen from the right ventricle, seems to be located beneath the pulmonary valve only, it is, like all other VSDs 'subaortic' when seen from the left ventricle, as the anomaly is due to absence of the infundibular septum, which is beneath the right aortic sinus in the left ventricular outflow tract. There is no ventricular septum above the aortic valve.

Inlet septal defects are described in detail with atrioventricular septal defects in Chapter 8. Small inlet septum VSDs sometimes occur in isolation, but most will, on close scrutiny, turn out to be extended perimembranous/malalignment VSDs (Figure 10.3a).

Trabecular septal VSDs are sometimes hidden beneath or anterior to the trabecula septomarginalis, and are thus difficult to see from the right ventricle. At the other end of the scale, the whole of the trabecular portion may be absent, so

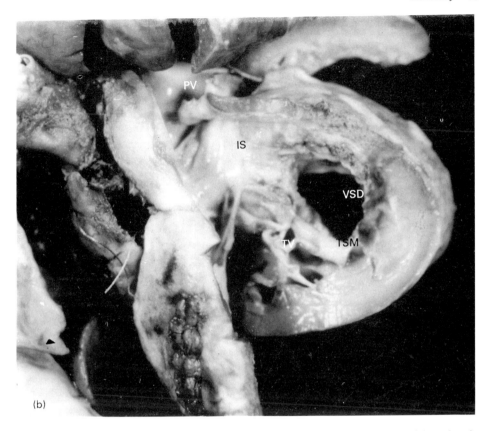

(b)

Figure 10.3 continued (b) Trabecular muscular VSD. This huge defect is due to absence of the trabecular septum, rather than the more common small defects among the trabeculae. IS, infundibular septum; PV, pulmonary valve; TSM, trabecula septomarginalis; TV, tricuspid valve

that the defect is huge (Figure 10.3b). Alternatively, there may be a mass of trabeculae at the apex with no septum at all, so that although at first sight there seems to be no VSD, probing will reveal that, on the contrary, there is no wall between the chambers.

Relationship of the VSD to the great arteries ('commitment')

Subarterial VSDs may lie directly beneath either the aorta or the pulmonary artery, so that the defect is said to be 'committed' to either artery. Similarly it may relate to both arteries (doubly committed) or to neither of them (uncommitted). Most isolated VSDs are located close to the aortic valve so that commitment is not significant, but it is an important determinant of haemodynamic and sometimes of anatomical status when discordant ventriculoarterial connections (e.g. double outlet right ventricle) are associated.

Acquired pulmonary outflow tract obstruction

Progressive hypertrophy of the trabecula septomarginalis and parietal trabeculae due to left-to-right shunting causes narrowing of the pulmonary infundibulum in a proportion of VSD hearts. It is morphologically distinct from the obstruction in tetralogy of Fallot (see Chapter 12), as there is no deviation of the infundibular septum: both ventricles become hypertrophied when the workload (pressure × flow) is increased by a big left-to-right shunt.

The earliest surgical management of VSD consisted of producing a degree of pulmonary outflow tract obstruction by partial ligation ('banding') of the pulmonary artery[4], and in the early days of cardiac surgery the operation electively preceded closure of the VSD. This strategy is obsolete for isolated VSD as the hospital mortality for primary closure in infants is now acceptably low. The two-stage operation is still used sometimes in the management of babies with multiple cardiac anomalies.

The operation

A discussion of the indications for operation is beyond the scope of this work, but is considered in detail elsewhere[5].

Most VSDs are accessible through either a right ventriculotomy or atriotomy, although some apical muscular defects are approached through a short left ventriculotomy between the distal segment of the anterior descending and diagonal branches of the left coronary artery. Both pulmonary arteriotomy and aortotomy have been used to approach the defect.

Small VSDs, particularly posterior muscular ones, may be closed by direct suture (interrupted and buttressed). Anteroapical defects are sometimes closed by bringing the sutures through the ventricular wall to the outside and tying them over felt pledgets.

Many perimembranous/malalignment and muscular defects can be closed through the tricuspid valve (right atriotomy) using a patch, while defects of the infundibular septum are usually closed through a short transverse incision in the infundibulum. This approach, rather than right atriotomy, may also be employed for perimembranous defects in infants.

Most surgeons use a Gore-Tex or a Dacron patch, although autologous pericardium, felt and felt faced with pericardium on the left ventricular aspect have all been used. The patch can be placed with either continuous or interrupted sutures.

If aortic regurgitation was present but mild, closure of the defect abolishes it. Moderate regurgitation may need plication of the aortic valve leaflets (through an aortotomy). Severe incompetence may necessitate valve replacement.

Pulmonary outflow tract obstruction is relieved through the ventriculotomy.

Necropsy

Early death

The risk of death in the immediate postoperative period is approximately 10–15% in babies under 6 months old[5], falling to around 5% for children between 6 months and 2 years old[5–7]. The risks are related directly to the patient's preoperative condition, which in turn reflects the degree of pulmonary hypertension. An excellent account of the microscopic anatomy of the pulmonary arteries in pulmonary hypertensive VSD is given by Wagenvoort *et al.*[8].

In infants, early death is likely to be associated with pulmonary complications.

Heart block
This is a rare complication but transient block may result when there is oedema in the region of the bundle. The depth of this structure in the myocardium is slightly variable so that the sutures may cause haemorrhage and/or oedema, bearing in mind that all the cardiac structures are small. If haemorrhage is not macroscopically visible it is advisable to examine the territory microscopically if this complication was suspected or known.

Incomplete closure
Like heartblock, this is a rare finding today, but the periphery of the patch should be probed to exclude the possibility. Also examine the septal surface from the left ventricle to exclude the possibility of a second VSD, although this is likely to have been diagnosed by 2D-echocardiography before operation.

Patent foramen ovale, ductus arteriosus
Even a trivial patency of the foramen ovale can permit a fatal intracardiac shunt in these haemodynamically precarious patients. The ductus closure should be examined meticulously to exclude the possibility that a ligature might have loosened.

Late death

Prolonged survival in these patients depends primarily upon the behaviour of the pulmonary vasculature so that the lungs are likely to offer more information than the heart itself. If the pulmonary vascular resistance was only mildly or moderately raised before operation, the prognosis is usually excellent if the operation was performed before the child was 2 years old. After that age about one-third develop pulmonary vascular disease. High preoperative pulmonary vascular resistance is generally associated with poor long-term results[5].

Infective endocarditis
The presence of the patch is a factor predisposing to infective endocarditis (see Chapter 4). Surgical revision of the patch is very seldom necessary and valve replacement is similarly uncommon. Endocarditis is a rare cause of late death.

Anticipated findings

1. Cardiac enlargement.
2. Healed incisions, right ventricular fibrosis associated with the ventriculotomy.
3. VSD patch: depending on how long the patient survived, the patch may be identifiable only by transilluminating the specimen. If it is obvious (i.e. not well healed or with areas not endothelialized), suspect either infective endocarditis or that there is a leak somewhere.

4. Primary closure of VSD is equally difficult to locate unless quite large pledgets were used. Careful palpation is the most reliable way to find them.
5. Jet lesions indicate a leak, but some endocardial thickening around the repair is usual and may be useful in pointing the way to (4) above.

Ventricular septal defect is a part of almost all the complex congenital anomalies, and much in the foregoing paragraphs applies to those as well as to the isolated anomaly.

References

1. Hoffman, J. I. E. Natural history of congenital heart disease. Problems in its assessment with special reference to ventricular septal defect. *Circulation,* **37**, 97–125, 1968
2. Allwork, S. P. and Anderson, R. H. The developmental anatomy of the membranous part of the ventricular septum. *British Heart Journal,* **41**, 275–280, 1979
3. Anderson, R. H., Becker, A. E. and van Mierop, L. H. S. What should we call the 'crista'? *British Heart Journal,* **39**, 856–959, 1977
4. Muller, W. H. Jr. and Dammann, J. F. Jr. Treatment of certain congenital malformations of the heart by the creation of pulmonic stenosis to relieve pulmonary hypertension and excessive pulmonary flow. A preliminary report. *Surgery, Gynecology and Obstetrics,* **95**, 213–219, 1952
5. Hoffman, J. I. E. and Rudolph, A. M. The natural history of isolated ventricular septal defect with special reference to selection of patients. *Advances in Pediatrics,* **17**, 57–79, 1970
6. Blackstone, E. H., Kirklin, J. W., Bradley, E. W. *et al.* Optimal age and results in repair of large ventricular septal defects. *Journal of Thoracic and Cardiovascular Surgery,* **72**, 661–679, 1976
7. Kirklin, J. W. and Dushane, J. W. Repair of ventricular septal defect in infancy. *Pediatrics,* **27**, 961–966, 1961
8. Wagenvoort, C. A., Neufeld, H. N., DuShane, J. W. and Edwards, J. E. The pulmonary arterial tree in ventricular septal defect. A quantitative study of anatomic features in fetuses, infants and children. *Circulation,* **23**, 740–748, 1961

11

Palliative operations

Many patients with complex congenital cardiac malformations have some surgical palliation before the radical operation is carried out. Although this book specifically concerns open rather than closed operations, a short section on these is given to facilitate the interpretation of the necropsy findings.

Operations to increase the blood supply to the lungs

Blalock–Taussig shunt (1944)[1]

In this operation the subclavian artery on the contralateral side to the aortic arch is approached through a lateral thoracotomy and anastomosed to the right or left pulmonary artery. Originally the operation was done in children and young adults, with good results. When the procedure was applied to babies the results were less good, as the subclavian artery is small in infants, so that it soon blocked due to low flow. This prompted the use of man-made grafts in babies ('modified' Blalock–Taussig operation).

Potts' anastomosis (1946)[2]

In this long-obsolete procedure the descending aorta was anastomosed to the left pulmonary artery via a left thoracotomy. The size of the stoma was difficult to control but was of vital importance to the fate of the vasculature of the left lung. In addition to problems concerned with the development of unilateral pulmonary hypertension, the stoma was difficult to close at the definitive operation and carried a high surgical mortality.

Brock's (closed) pulmonary valvotomy (1948)[3]

The original approach for this operation was a left anterolateral thoracotomy. A dilator, most descriptively called a 'cobra-head', was introduced through the apex of the right ventricle via a controlled stab wound and passed several times through the stenotic pulmonary valve. Like the Blalock–Taussig operation, this procedure was designed for children, not babies, in whom the structures are small and delicate and who may have a significant shunt through a patent foramen ovale.

This closed procedure has long been superseded by open pulmonary valvotomy, and is hardly ever performed in babies now; adult patients may carry the surgical scar.

Brock's (closed) pulmonary infundibulectomy (1950)[4]

Like the valvotomy this operation is now usually done 'open', and thus under direct vision. Originally the right ventricle was approached as above, and an instrument ending in two apposable 'spoons' with sharpened edges was introduced into the narrowed infundibulum. Several grams of muscle could be removed and the results immediately assessed by pressure measurements.

Waterston's anastomosis (1962)[5]

In this procedure the heart is approached through a median sternotomy, the pericardium opened and the ascending aorta anastomosed to the right pulmonary artery.

Although the stoma size may present difficulties (too big or too small), and the right pulmonary artery may become 'tented' and thus occluded as the child grows, this operation, together with the 'modified' Blalock–Taussig procedure is the operation probably most commonly used today for the palliation of severe pulmonary outflow tract obstruction in infants preparatory to radical operation. The Waterston anastomosis is less hazardous to take down at the definitive operation than the Pott's. (In the USA this procedure is sometimes called a Waterston–Cooley shunt. Independently of Waterston, Cooley devised the operation and described it in an American journal[6]. Waterston's publication antedated this by 4 years).

Operations to reduce the flow to the lungs

The only operation in this group is that of partial ligation of the main pulmonary artery. The procedure is known as 'banding' and was introduced in 1952[7]. It was the first form of surgical therapy for ventricular septal defect (see Chapter 10).

Operations to bypass the right side of the heart

Glenn's operation (1954)[8]

This operation, in which the superior vena cava is anastomosed to the right pulmonary artery, is only very rarely used to palliate malformations in which pulmonary outflow tract obstruction is life threatening. One reason is that when radical operation is to come, it is made very difficult by the presence of a Glenn shunt. The procedure was the operation of choice for tricuspid atresia before the introduction of Fontan's operation.

Fontan's operation (1971)[9]

This complex operation was devised for the treatment of tricuspid atresia but is also done to palliate other congenital cardiac malformations by means of bypassing the right side of the heart.

The superior vena cava is anastomosed end-to-side to the right pulmonary artery. The right atrial appendage is anastomosed by means of a conduit (with or without a bioprosthetic valve) to the proximal stump of the right pulmonary artery. The interatrial communication is closed and another bioprosthetic valve is placed in the inferior vena cava. Lastly, the superior vena cava is divided below the first anastomosis and the closure of the two ends.

There have been several modifications to the procedure so that there may be but one valve (either inlet or outlet) or none.

Bjork's operation (1979)[10]

The right atrial appendage is anastomosed to the right ventricle, using a pericardial patch graft. It can be done only when the right ventricle is capable of pumping (i.e. not too underdeveloped). This simple procedure does not employ a valve, so that repeated replacement is avoided. However, the 'subpulmonary chamber' is not considered beneficial nowadays, and the use of magnification, together with improved monofilament suture materials, permits adequate palliation by other means.

References

1. Blalock, A. and Taussig, H. B. The surgical treatment of the heart in which there is either pulmonary stenosis or pulmonary atresia. *Journal of the American Medical Association,* **128,** 189–202, 1945
2. Potts, J. W., Smith, S. and Gibson, S. Anastomosis of the aorta to a pulmonary artery. *Journal of the American Medical Association,* **132,** 627–631, 1946
3. Brock, R. C. Pulmonary valvulotomy for the relief of congenital pulmonary stenosis. Report of three cases. *British Medical Journal,* **1,** 1121–1126, 1948
4. Brock, R. C. and Campbell, M. Infundibular resection for pulmonic stenosis. *British Heart Journal,* **12,** 403–424, 1950
5. Waterston, D. J. Treatment of Fallot's tetralogy in children under one year of age. *Rozhledy v Chirugii,* **41,** 181–183, 1962
6. Cooley, D. A. and Hallman, D. G. Intrapericardial aortic–right pulmonary arterial shunt. *Surgery, Gynecology and Obstetrics,* **122,** 1084–1086, 1966
7. Muller, W. H. Jr. and Dammann, J. F. Jr. Treatment of certain congenital malformations of the heart by the creation of pulmonic stenosis to relieve pulmonary hypertension and excessive pulmonary flow. *Surgery, Gynecology and Obstetrics,* **95,** 213–219, 1952
8. Glenn, W. W. L. Circulatory bypass of the right side of the heart. Intervenous shunt between the superior vena cava and the distal right pulmonary artery. *New England Journal of Medicine,* **259,** 117–120, 1958
9. Fontan, F. and Baudet, E. Surgical repair of tricuspid atresia. *Thorax,* **26,** 240–248, 1971
10. Bjork, V. O., Olin, C. L., Bjarke, B. B. and Thoren, C. A. Right atrial–right ventricular anastomosis for correction of tricuspid atresia. *Journal of Thoracic and Cardiovascular Surgery,* **77,** 452–458, 1979

12

Tetralogy of Fallot

The haemodynamic status determines the severity of the illness in any given patient, while the anatomical arrangements determine the ease or otherwise of the surgical operation.

Fallot was not the first to recognize this common malformation, but it was he who first applied the noun 'tetralogy' to the well-known complex of:

- Infundibular pulmonary outflow tract obstruction
- Ventricular septal defect (VSD)
- Overriding (dextroposition) of the aorta
- Right ventricular hypertrophy[1,2].

The pathognomonic features are the first two; the position of the aorta relative to the pulmonary artery and the VSD depends upon the type of VSD (e.g. muscular infundibular, perimembranous/malalignment, etc.) and the degree of hypoplasia of the pulmonary outflow tract, while the hypertrophy reflects the left-to-right shunt and is biventricular. Many patients also have a persistently patent foramen ovale or an ASD. Persistence of the ductus arteriosus, even in infants, is, however, uncommon.

In the early days of surgical cardiology, many patients with VSD and pulmonary outflow tract obstruction due to other malformations were categorized as having Fallot's tetralogy, and, if they were atypical, e.g. with a large heart in the absence of heart failure, they were described as Fallot variants. There is a limited range of morphological variance in this malformation, and an aphorism, 'if it's not obviously Fallot's tetralogy, then it's obviously not', is most applicable to the disorder. Fallot's tetralogy is a specific type of pulmonary outflow tract malformation obligatorily coupled with a large VSD. All hearts with tetralogy of Fallot have this specific anatomy, but by no means all hearts with VSD and pulmonary outflow tract obstruction have Fallot's tetralogy.

The *pulmonary outflow tract obstruction* is always at least partly due to anterior deviation of the indundibular septum which causes unequal division of the aortic and pulmonary outflow tracts at the expense of the latter. This obstruction may be aggravated by any or all of the following:

- Hypertrophy of parietal trabeculae
- High origin of the trabecula septomarginalis (sometimes called the 'moderator band')
- A combination of these to produce multiple sites of obstruction, sometimes resulting in a 'two-chambered right ventricle'[3,4].

Very rarely the pulmonary outflow tract is further obstructed by aneurysm of the membranous part of the ventricular septum.

Pulmonary valve stenosis co-exists in many cases, so that there is both valvular and infundibular stenosis. Rarely, the pulmonary valve is absent. In this disorder the pulmonary trunk is dilated but branch stenoses are present. The outflow tract narrowing does, however, correspond to that in Fallot's tetralogy, so that they are classified together.

Irrespective of associated valvular stenosis, the infundibular obstruction in Fallot's tetralogy is progressive, as platelets and fibrin are deposited just below the valve, while progressive right ventricular hypertrophy augments the anatomical abnormalities.

The *VSD* in Fallot's tetralogy is *always* large, having at least the diameter of the aortic valve, or more. In case-notes it is often described, rather unhelpfully, as 'high', and, even more unhelpfully, as 'being in the usual place'. The high position indicates that the defect is related to the aortic valve, which overrides it to a variable degree, but the VSD itself may be of any kind (see below).

Associated muscular VSDs are uncommon in Fallot's tetralogy and, if present, are an additional malformation: the subaortic VSD is an integral part of the developmental anomaly. The VSD is *never* 'restrictive' in Fallot's tetralogy. Restrictive VSD together with pulmonary outflow tract obstruction is a different malformation.

As in isolated VSD, the defect may be of the perimembranous/malalignment type, or it may be of the infundibular muscular kind. More than two-thirds of all Fallot VSDs are in one of these two categories. Often the defect extends to embrace both the membranous and muscular parts of the septum. In the third, less common type, the infundibular septum is absent so that the defect extends anteriorly to the pulmonary valve. (In view of the remarks above about anterior deviation of the infundibular septum being the hallmark of the anomaly, it may be argued that hearts with this anatomy are not morphologically 'Fallot hearts'. However, their physiological behaviour is indistinguishable from the others, and the only way in which they *may* differ from them is that they form a substantial proportion of the patients who are not cyanosed at rest, or who do not develop cyanosis until adult life, the so-called 'acyanotic tetralogy of Fallot'.)

Atrioventricular septal defect associated with the tetralogy of Fallot is particularly associated with patients with trisomy 21 (so-called Down's syndrome).

The *aortic override* varies from negligible to 100%. Appreciation of the degree of override is important to the surgeon, as it may determine the surgical strategy for a given patient. If more than 50% of the aortic valve originates from the right ventricle, double outlet right ventricle (DORV) is present. As this is usually deduced by angiography or 2D-echocardiography in the preoperative period, it often denotes a relationship rather than an anatomical connection. However, 'anatomical' DORV does coexist with Fallot's tetralogy.

It is not necessary to be able to demonstrate loss of fibrous continuity between the aortic and mitral valves to identify the abnormal connection (DORV) in this malformation.

The operation

The surgical mortality is about 5% or less, particularly for patients over a year old[5]. The major determinants of surgical outcome are the size of the pulmonary artery and/or the status of the blood supply to the lungs.

Any palliative procedures are taken down at the radical operation. Systemic–pulmonary collateral channels are ligated. It is feasible to embolize collateral vessels prior to the thoracotomy, but, if the patient is dependent upon them, obviously some must be retained until then. This additional procedure increases the risk of surgical mortality.

The VSD is almost always patched, even in babies. The patch is placed with either interrupted or continuous suture.

The pulmonary outflow tract is treated by direct resection if possible. Parietal trabeculae can be excised and the free wall may be thinned. Valvular stenosis is relieved under direct vision. If the main pulmonary artery is hypoplastic and/or the outflow tract is not amenable to direct resection, an outflow tract patch may be necessary. This can be placed below the pulmonary valve as a gusset (rarely done nowadays), or carried across the annulus of the pulmonary valve to the bifurcation of the pulmonary artery (transannular patch). These patches may be of autologous or heterologous pericardium, Dacron, or a composite graft of one of these materials. Alternatively, a single allograft aortic leaflet and sinus, often with the anterior mitral leaflet attached, to give anchorage to the sutures may be chosen. This last type of graft is often called 'monocusp'.

The foregoing paragraphs give no indication of the often complex and difficult nature of the operation, but the necropsy findings sometimes reflect them.

Necropsy

Early death

When patients, particularly babies, die in the early postoperative period the necropsy findings may seem to be unable to account for the death. Several apparently trivial things, such as a minute residual patency of a previous palliative shunt, may have a cumulative effect on these patients in critical haemodynamic balance.

Fallot's tetralogy is a 'small heart' malformation so that a heavy heart is indicative of oedema. A large heart should alert one to the possibility of a different anatomical diagnosis except in the (very rare nowadays) adult patients coming to operation in terminal heart failure.

Haemorrhage
This is a less common cause of fatality than it used to be, but is still a major factor in patients with long-standing palliative procedures and those with multiple collateral channels.

Previous operations
The site of a previous Blalock shunt is quite difficult to find at necropsy, and is *impossible* if the heart and lungs have been separated. The subclavian artery is a small vessel in babies and does not grow much when used for this purpose, so that there is a tendency for it to atrophy. Similarly, a Waterston site can be hard to assess as it is intrapericardial and may be obscured by oedema and haemorrhage. As patch repair and enlargement of the pulmonary artery is often necessary, location of this patch is helpful in identifying the site.

Intracardiac shunts
There are two main causes of intracardiac shunts in the early postoperative period:

1. *Interatrial communication*: many Fallot patients have a patent foramen ovale, and if it is small it may be ignored or overlooked at operation. In these haemodynamically unstable patients, even a tiny hole can permit a fatal shunt. Careful examination of the atrial septum is mandatory in these cases to locate such a potential for catastrophe.
2. *Interventricular communication*: with contemporary cardioplegic techniques incomplete closure of the VSD is very uncommon but occasionally a suture or suture line gives way. This is more likely to occur when a continuous suture was used, as, when the heart is flaccid under cardioplegia, it is possible to put too

much tension on the monofilament. If continuous suture is used, the patch is applied with at least two lengths, so that it never completely gives way. Interrupted sutures rarely cut out, and if they do, they leave but a small gap.

Iatrogenic VSD
This rare complication results from muscle resection on or close to the septal surface when parietal trabeculae were resected. It may manifest during the first postoperative hours if the resection was extensive, but is more likely to occur at 10–12 days after operation, due to myocardial necrosis. The appearance is similar to that of ischaemic VSD in coronary artery disease, but the lesion is located (usually) near the anteroapical section of the VSD patch.

Removal of the patch   It is usually easier to see the VSD and identify its type if the patch is taken out after assessment of the repair. Using small curved scissors, cut close to each knot on the right ventricular aspect: after a few sutures have been cut, the remainder of the removal is much facilitated by using dissecting forceps as well. Forceps are not recommended at the beginning as it is quite easy to damage the boundaries of the repair.

Note. If removal of the VSD patch is undesirable for any reason, the type of VSD (perimembranous/malalignment, infundibular muscular, absent infundibular septum) can be identified by transilluminating the region of the defect. As in isolated VSD, perimembranous VSDs have a fibrous posterior boundary, formed by the fibrous continuity linking the tricuspid, aortic and mitral valves via the membranous septum. The remainder all have a muscular posterior boundary, and the membranous septum will clearly be seen posterior to the VSD, irrespective of whether the heart is transilluminated from either the left or the right ventricle.

Extracardiac shunts
Palliative shunts tend to close spontaneously and are often not demonstrable at preoperative assessment. Modified Blalock shunts, in particular, become occluded by concentric development of fibrointimal hyperplasia. If no flow was demonstrable during preoperative study the shunt is likely to be left alone, as taking it down can be hazardous. However, the conduit may remain minutely (but macroscopically) patent, so that flow may become significant in the haemodynamically disturbed postoperative period.

Systemic–pulmonary collateral arteries
These vessels are sometimes erroneously called 'bronchial arteries'. The paired bronchial arteries arise a few millimetres distal to the left subclavian artery as the first branches of the descending aorta. They pass along the superior border of the bronchi and branch with them. They are recognized microscopically by their close relationship to the bronchi and bronchioles. Although they sometimes become greatly enlarged in pulmonary outflow tract obstruction, they are morphologically distinct from the systemic–pulmonary collateral arteries which arise, usually unpaired, from the descending aorta. These vessels are reopened or redeveloped intersegmental arteries and pass into the lung parenchyma in a random fashion. They do not accompany the bronchi, pulmonary arteries or veins, but they do anastomose freely with the arteries.

Although it is feasible to embolize many of these collateral arteries under radiological control prior to the surgical operation, some may have to be left until then. They are not always easy to identify at operation, and as they are generally inaccessible through a median sternotomy, some may be missed. Like the surgically placed shunts, they may deliver a significant flow after operation. Furthermore, the dissection to locate and tie them can be a major source of bleeding.

Conduction disturbance

Contrary to often expressed opinion, iatrogenic heart block is, and always has been, an extremely rare occurrence. In 30 years in a Cardiothoracic Unit, the author can recall only two patients who needed permanent pacemakers; both occurred in the late 1950s.

The common bundle is potentially at risk *only* in perimembranous/malalignment VSD (i.e. in only about a third of cases) in which the membranous septum forms the posterior boundary of the defect. However, the right bundle branch sometimes takes a superficial course in this anomaly and does not 'leave' the border of the defect until it reaches the infundibular papillary muscle of the tricuspid valve. Iatrogenic damage may occur to the right bundle branch, but is usually non-contributory to the fatality.

As in isolated perimembranous VSD, the common bundle may be unusually superficial, and temporary arrythmias can result from haemorrhage and oedema in the region of the bundle. If present, the haemorrhagic area is usually obvious at necropsy, and tedious serial sectioning of the bundle is unnecessary. If damage to the conducting system was suspected, careful removal of the patch by cutting the sutures will reveal the summit of the septum, from which a block can be taken.

Degree of aortic override

In most cases assessment of the ventriculoarterial connection (normal or double outlet right ventricle) presents no problems at all. However, there are those in which it may be uncertain. For example, the 2D-echocardiography and/or the angiocardiogram suggest a DORV connection, while the operation findings disagree.

DORV in association with Fallot's tetralogy is a slightly contentious matter. According to one author[6], Fallot's tetralogy and DORV are separate entities which may co-exist, while others[7] claim that the loss of the normal ventriculoarterial connection expressed as DORV with Fallot's tetralogy represents one end of the spectrum of the malformation.

Fallot's tetralogy is a specific kind of malalignment of the infundibular septum, while DORV is a ventriculoarterial connection, so that there should be no intellectual difficulties in reconciling the two. The recognition of DORV is often subjective, as it is often expressed as a relationship rather than a connection, and dependent upon the observer's position (e.g. a beating heart at operation versus a fixed, dead one).

In most hearts with Fallot's tetralogy the superior aspect of the VSD is the aortic valve. Permembranous/malalignment VSDs lie between the limbs of the trabecula septomarginalis so that there is aorto-mitral-tricuspid fibrous continuity. Infundibular muscular VSDs are also roofed by the aortic valve leaflets, and also lie between the limbs of the trabecula septomarginalis, but because the inferior limb of the trabecula septomarginalis is continuous with the ventriculoinfundibular fold, the posterior boundary of the defect is muscular, not fibrous. However, the normal aortomitral continuity is retained by the (normal) membranous part of the ventricular septum. Thus, it is unnecessary to 'require' the absence of mitral-aortic fibrous continuity to diagnose DORV in a heart with Fallot's tetralogy. If only a little over half of the aortic valve overrides, there is Fallot's tetralogy with DORV, while, if the aorta originates exclusively from the right ventricle in the presence of the pathognomonic infundibular malformation of Fallot's tetralogy, then it is appropriate to classify the heart as DORV with Fallot's tetralogy.

Note. It is virtually impossible to determine the ventriculoarterial connection if the unfixed heart is opened by cutting through the aortic and pulmonary outflow tracts. It is completely impossible if more than one cut is made through each artery! If the dissection has to be completed on the fresh specimen, cutting through the aortic valve from the left ventricular side should be avoided, as it is this, in particular, which destroys the anatomy and makes the connection so difficult to recognize.

Ideally, open the fixed right ventricle through the tricuspid valve at the acute margin and continue to the apex. In the larger hearts this usually gives an adequate view of the VSD and resected outflow tract, so that the ventriculoarterial connection can be identified after taking out the patch. In smaller hearts it will almost certainly be necessary to continue the incision from the apex to just below the pulmonary valve. It should now be possible to see the nature of the connection. If there is an outflow tract patch, continue the cut through the middle of it, but without prejudice to its own status, to display the outflow tract. If possible, leave this part of the dissection until the last so that the patches in both the VSD and the outflow tract have already been examined.

Right ventricular hypertrophy

As previously stated, there is biventricular hypertrophy in most cases. While the walls of the right ventricle are thick, the chamber itself is often small, and may further be diminished by the VSD patch, the outflow tract patch (if present) and the closure of the ventriculotomy. This may be a contributory cause in early postoperative deaths (although the author has no scientific evidence to support this view). Not only is the right ventricular cavity small, but its thick walls have an abundance of fibrous tissue, even in babyhood. When the contractile properties of the already compromised ventricular wall are further inhibited by the operation, it seems likely that right ventricular function may be impaired.

Coronary artery 'anomalies'

Up to 5% of hearts with Fallot's tetralogy have some variant of coronary artery anatomy. The most usual one is origin of the anterior descending branch from the right coronary artery rather than the left [8]. Another common finding is that of the right coronary artery passing anterior to the pulmonary valve, thus forming part of the pulmonary outflow tract. This, together with prominent right ventricular branches, is a fairly common finding in all congenital cardiac malformations which include pulmonary outflow tract obstruction [9].

Obviously, the major epicardial branches are plainly visible at a first operation, but many patients have undergone previous intrapericardial operations. Many surgeons make a diagram of the coronary anatomy, and today coronary arteriography is feasible even in infants, so that major mishaps are rare. However, smaller right ventricular branches may be overlooked, and accidental transection of such apparently minor arteries may produce a disproportionately large area of myocardial necrosis at around 10–12 days after operation. This complication exacerbates those outlined in the preceding remarks on the right ventricle.

It is stressed that although variations in coronary artery anatomy are fairly common in Fallot's tetralogy, complications due to the coronary arteries are extremely rare.

Late death

Unlike patients with isolated VSD, long-term survival is not dependent upon changes in the pulmonary vascular bed. Instead, it depends primarily upon a satisfactory haemodynamic result having been achieved at operation, and subsequently upon freedom from infective endocarditis (like all cardiac surgical patients, irrespective of disease), together with non-recurrence of either VSD or pulmonary outflow tract obstruction, and absence of fatal arrythmias. Reoperation for any of these is hazardous and carries a significant mortality.

In sharp contrast to early deaths, the heart late after radical operation for Fallot's tetralogy is enlarged, and the right ventricle may still predominate. As in all late deaths, the atrial appendages may not be apparent at first sight, and ventriculotomy and left ventricular vent scars may be visible once the pericardium is removed. Similarly, outflow tract enlargement with a cloth patch may be visible.

Residual/recurrent pulmonary outflow tract obstruction

Because the obstruction may have been multifocal, it may not always have been possible completely to extirpate it at operation, especially where parietal trabeculae were responsible. Muscular obstruction may recur, either relatively early (within a year or so) or late (up to 20 years). Valvular stenosis can recur as well, particularly when a less than optimal fall in right ventricular pressure was obtained at operation.

The appearance of this 'new' obstruction is variable. There is often quite marked endocardial thickening, which is patchy, indicating turbulence. The stumps of resected muscle bands are fibrotic, and enlarged (unlike amputated mitral papillary muscles which atrophy after valve replacement). Anticipated sites for this are the tricuspid papillary muscles themselves, the site of origin of the trabecula septomarginalis, and the distal part of the outflow tract.

The pulmonary valve is also variable in appearance, but the variation usually reflects the degree of derangement rather than a range of morphology. It may be possible to discern whether the valve is bicuspid or tricuspid, but seldom is, as the sinuses are but poorly developed and the leaflets may be so deformed and thickened. The leaflets are often shrunken and re-fused, and the resulting immobility is aggravated by calcification.

If a transannular patch was used, there is obligatory pulmonary valve regurgitation and the leaflet morphology is difficult to discern. Sometimes leaflets may be represented by no more than verrucous elevations in the pulmonary artery. If a single leaflet allograft was used to lessen the regurgitation, calcification of the implanted aortic wall is anticipated, together with degeneration of the leaflet, as in other allograft valve replacements.

Because there is often pulmonary valve regurgitation with consequent dilatation of the right ventricle, thickening and hooding of the *tricuspid* valve leaflets occur with some frequency. In older patients this may also be associated with calcification of the leaflets, and, more rarely, of part of the tricuspid annulus.

Aneurysmal dilatation of the main pulmonary artery
This is associated with both transannular patches and with allograft enlargement of the pulmonary outflow tract. Unlike the funnel-shaped poststenotic dilatation, the aneurysms are discrete, and may be quite large. Spontaneous rupture is rare.

The VSD patch
In very late deaths the presence of the patch may be inferred only by a few tell-tale suture ends. In patients operated upon in the 1950s and early 1960s, when silk was the only suture material available, these ends may be easy to see, but the newer monofilament materials give themselves away less easily. It is most helpful to be able to transilluminate the septum to locate a really well-healed patch and to discriminate between it and the membranous part of the ventricular septum.

Residual VSD is very uncommon nowadays, due to the better access which modern cardioplegic techniques afford, but infective endocarditis may cause disruption to the VSD repair, even many years later.

Arrythmias
Late death in operated Fallot's tetralogy is often sudden and unexpected, and postexertional deaths are relatively common in adults. While many such deaths are explicable because of pulmonary outflow tract obstruction, etc., a great many patients have clinically significant conduction disturbances.

The occurrence of postoperative arrythmias, especially right bundle branch block, is at least in part linked to the patient's age at operation, and also to the surgical technique employed for closing the VSD. Right bundle branch block occurs in those over 8 years of age at operation, and also in a high proportion of those who had a large right ventriculotomy.

Supraventricular tachycardia is present in a proportion of patients, who may succumb despite treatment with antiarrhythmic drugs, but the more common conduction disturbances are confined to the peripheral conducting system, so that they are expressed as left anterior hemiblock, or, less commonly, bifascicular block.

Menacing ventricular tachycardias are associated with fibrosis of the right ventricle, subsequent to ventriculotomy, and these behave in a manner similar to left ventricular arrythmias due to infarction.

It is emphasized that arrythmias associated with the proximal conducting system are extremely rare: fibrosis of the common bundle does not occur (after all, it was potentially at risk during operation in only a third of patients initially), but minute foci of fibrosis associated with patch sutures may play a part in aggravating arrythmias in right ventricles which from birth had more fibrous tissue than those of normal individuals. Thinning and marked fibrosis are characteristic of the anterior wall of the right ventricle in these patients. Ventricular arrythmias associated with this are analogous to postinfarction arrythmias in the left ventricle in ischaemic heart disease.

Coronary artery disease
Radical operation of a congenital malformation does not, of course, confer any immunity to ischaemic heart disease in later life. At least one patient in the Hammersmith series has returned after an interval of 22 years for bypass grafts to diseased coronary arteries. In older patients, coronary artery disease is at least as likely a cause of death as arrythmia, and is a great deal easier to identify.

Summary

The anticipated findings in late death after operation for Fallot's tetralogy are:

1. Enlarged heart (usually).
2. Endocardial thickening of right ventricle.
3. Dilatation of right ventricle, sometimes causing:
4. (Tricuspid valve regurgitation.)
5. Small pulmonary trunk, or
6. Surgical augmentation of the pulmonary outflow tract.
7. VSD patch (rarely, residual/recurrent VSD).
8. Abnormal pulmonary valve or allograft replacement or outflow tract patch.
9. (Coronary artery disease, myocardial infarction.)
10. (Identifiable pathology of the conducting system.)

References

1. Fallot, E. L. A. Contribution à l'anatomie pathologique de la maladie bleue (cyanose cardiaque). *Marseille Médicale, 25,* 77–93, 1888
2. Allwork, S. P. Tetralogy of Fallot: the centenary of the name. (A new translation of the first of Fallot's papers.) *European Journal of Cardiothoracic Surgery, 2,* 386–392, 1988
3. Anderson, R. H., Allwork, S. P., Ho, S. Y. *et al.* Surgical anatomy of the tetralogy of Fallot. *Journal of Thoracic and Cardiovascular Surgery, 81,* 887–896, 1981
4. Restivo, A., Cameron, A. H., Anderson, R. H. and Allwork, S. P. Divided right ventricle: a review of the anatomical varieties. *Pediatric Cardiology, 5,* 197–204, 1984
5. Kirklin, J. W., Blackstone, E. H. and Pacifico, A. D. Routine primary repair vs. two-stage repair of tetralogy of Fallot. *Circulation, 60,* 373–386, 1979
6. Edwards, W. D. Double outlet right ventricle and tetralogy of Fallot; two distinct but not mutually exclusive entities. *Journal of Thoracic and Cardiovascular Surgery, 82,* 418–422, 1981
7. Wilcox, B. R., Ho, S. Y., Macartney, F. J. *et al.* Surgical anatomy of double outlet right ventricle with situs solitus and atrioventricular concordance. *Journal of Thoracic and Cardiovascular Surgery, 82,* 268–271, 1981
8. Fellows, K. E., Freed, M. D., Keane, J. F. *et al.* Results of routine preoperative coronary angiography in tetralogy of Fallot. *Circulation, 51,* 561–566, 1975
9. Allwork, S. P. The anatomy of the outflow tracts of the heart and of aortic and pulmonary allografts. In *Cardiac Valve Allografts 1962–1987* (eds A. C. Yankah *et al.*), Steinkopff-Verlag, Darmstadt, pp. 107–111, 1988

13

Transposition of the aorta and pulmonary artery

Transposition of the aorta and pulmonary artery is an abnormality of ventriculoarterial connection which is nearly always associated with abnormal interrelationship of the great arteries. It is emphasized that the disorder is *not* the positional anomaly itself.

The malformation, which has been recognized since the early eighteenth century, is given several names: for example, 'transposition of the great arteries', often abbreviated to TGA; 'transposition of the great vessels' (TGV), which is unsatisfactory, as only the arteries are involved; and, perhaps most accurately, 'ventriculoarterial discordance'.

Ventriculoarterial discordance is that condition in which the aorta arises exclusively from the *morphological* right ventricle, and the pulmonary artery arises exclusively from the *morphological* left ventricle. From this, it is evident that malpositions of the aorta such as double outlet right ventricle or single outlet heart (e.g. so-called pulmonary atresia) are not forms of transposition, as they have sometimes been described. For transposition to be present, both arteries must be placed across (i.e. transposed) the ventricular septum. Positional anomalies of the aorta and pulmonary artery *without* this discordant ventriculoarterial connection are called malpositions of the arteries. The positional interrelationship, e.g. aorta anterior and to the right, is expressed in that manner. Anterior aorta does *not* equal arterial transposition.

From the definition above, it is a simple matter to identify and describe the morbid anatomy of the heart in this anomaly without the necessity of resorting to physiological or spatial nomenclature, which serve only to confuse in this context. Description is further simplified if it is remembered that the atrioventricular valves *and* the coronary arteries accord with the ventricles, irrespective of the spatial arrangement or the position of the heart in the chest, or the location of the apex of the heart.

Anatomy

The atria have normally-connected veins, but left superior vena cava is found in a proportion of cases. Natural interatrial communications are quite frequent, but as most patients are palliated in the first day or two of life by balloon septostomy (Rashkind's procedure, see below), almost all have, at best, a large round hole in the atrial septum and, less optimally, a tear in the fossa ovalis. Atrioventricular concordance is present; the right atrium is connected by a tricuspid valve to a morphologically right ventricle. Commonly, the ventricular septum is intact (no VSD), and the infundibulum of the right ventricle gives origin to the aorta. The left atrium is connected to the left ventricle by a mitral valve. The pulmonary valve originates from the left ventricle in fibrous continuity with the mitral valve.

This basic arrangement is often called simple transposition, and refers to the absence of a VSD. An occasional feature in simple transposition is a disproportion between the inlet and outlet lengths of the ventricular septum, similar to that seen in AVSD, but without the valve anomalies and without the AVSD. The ventricular septum is straighter than in the normal heart and the interventricular portion of the membranous septum is usually absent.

Externally, the aorta and pulmonary artery have a rather variable interrelationship. The aorta may be directly anterior to the pulmonary artery, slightly obliquely anterior, or alongside it (often called side-by-side arteries). The arteries ascend together without crossing. It is this detail of adult morphology which has stimulated interest and controversy about the developmental origin of the malformation for the last hundred years or so.

Coronary artery anatomy

The origin and disposition of the coronary arteries is, as might be anticipated, variable in this malformation. In almost all cases, as in the normal heart, the two coronary arteries originate in one or both of the aortic sinuses which face the pulmonary valve, so that the origin of the arteries is dependent upon the interrelationship of the aorta and the pulmonary artery, e.g. side-by-side, anteroposterior. Thus, in hearts in which the aorta is directly anterior to the pulmonary artery, the coronary arteries originate in the two posterior sinuses, while the most anterior sinus is 'non-coronary'. In side-by-side arteries the coronary ostia are situated in the posterior and left anterior sinuses and the right anterior sinus is the non-coronary sinus.

Single coronary artery is an uncommon finding in ventriculoarterial discordance.

The branching pattern of the coronary arteries is also partly dependent upon the arterial interrelationship and upon the presence of a VSD. In over 60% of cases the left coronary artery has its ostium in the more anterior of the two facing aortic sinuses, while the right coronary artery originates in the posterior facing sinus. In simple transposition the arteries usually ramify in a manner comparable with that in the normal heart, but where a VSD is present the branching pattern is likely to be deranged.

Classification of the variants of coronary artery anatomy in transposition is complicated by the spatial anomalies; several classifications have been offered, but are confusing. A clear, comprehensible account and system for classification is given by Gittenberger de Groot et al. and by Sauer et al. [1,2].

Associated anomalies

Ventricular septal defect

The most commonly associated anomaly in arterial transposition is VSD and the defect may be of any kind. Malalignment VSDs may be straddled by tensor apparatus from the mitral valve. Where the aorta is left-sided, either valve can straddle.

As in normal hearts, the ventricles are of equal wall thickness at birth, but even in the presence of a VSD that of the left regresses by the age of 8 months.

Pulmonary outflow tract obstruction

When the ventricular septum is intact, pulmonary outflow tract obstruction corresponds to that of aortic outflow tract obstruction in ventriculoarterial concordance, i.e. it can be valvular or subvalvular, dynamic or fixed.

Pulmonary outflow tract obstruction in transposition with VSD has a poor prognosis and the nature of the obstruction differs from that in simple transposition. The obstruction may be due to a deviated infundibular septum bulging into the left ventricular outflow tract. Other causes are aneurysm of the poorly developed interventricular part of the membranous septum and anomalous attachment of mitral chordae tendineae.

Patent ductus arteriosus

This occurs with some frequency beyond babyhood, and coarctation of the aorta and interrupted aortic arch may also be present.

Collateral circulation

Large, often bilateral, collateral arteries are to be found passing to the lungs from the descending aorta. These vessels act as a naturally occurring bypass, and may vascularize a considerable amount of lung tissue (Figure 13.1). These vessels are not a constant finding in TGA, but may be haemodynamically significant when present.

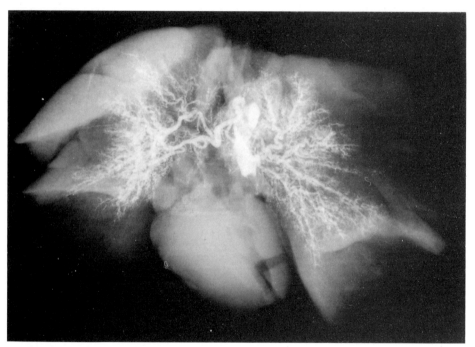

Figure 13.1 Post-mortem arteriogram of extensive major aorticopulmonary collateral arteries (MAPCAs) in a baby with TGA. These MAPCAs may permit a significant shunt in the absence of intracardiac shunts or outflow tract obstruction, and occur with some frequency in ventriculoarterial discordance

Operations

From the foregoing it is obvious that unless there is some possibility, either natural or iatrogenic, for the systemic and pulmonary circulations to mix, the malformation is incompatible with extrauterine life.

The first operation to palliate the anomaly was surgical excision of the atrial septum, introduced by Blalock and Hanlon in 1950[3]. The introduction of the balloon septostomy by Rashkind and Miller in 1966[4] has rendered the surgical operation largely obsolete, and most babies now undergo the latter during the diagnostic study in the first day or two of life. It has the disadvantage of often producing only a small hole, so further treatment is necessary earlier than when surgical excision was done.

The earliest open operation was outlined in principle by Mustard in 1954[5]. The inferior vena cava flow was rerouted to the left atrium and the right pulmonary venous return to the left atrium. The operation was first performed successfully by Baffes in 1956[6].

The first successful correction at atrial level was achieved in 1959 by Senning[7] and is in use today. All the venous return is rerouted by constructing a systemic venous atrium from the anterior part of the left atrium and the posterior part of the right, augmenting with autologous pericardium where necessary. Pulmonary venous return is directed to the right ventricle by anastomosing the posterior part of the left atrium to the anterior part of the right. In this procedure there is no prosthetic material inside the heart.

In 1964, Mustard[8] introduced the procedure which bears his name. The atria are reapportioned by means of a baffle of pericardium or man-made prosthetic material. The atrial septum is excised and the patch, shaped like trousers, is placed with the waist under the pulmonary veins and the free wall of the left atrium, while the legs are sewn around the openings of the two venae cavae and the crotch is secured to the remnant of the atrial septum.

Rastelli[9] in 1969 devised a procedure for transposition with VSD. The VSD is used to form part of a tunnel of prosthetic material to connect the aorta to the left ventricle. A valved conduit connects the right ventricle to the pulmonary trunk, the pulmonary valve having been oversewn before transecting or incising the pulmonary artery.

The operation of McGoon[10] requires the presence of a large VSD, as a boomerang-shaped patch is placed in such a manner that the left ventricle empties into the aorta via the VSD while the right ventricle communicates with the pulmonary artery.

None of these operations is curative, and the last two are suitable only for older patients who also have the disadvantage of the thin-walled left ventricle. Anatomical, true correction of the malformation was achieved by Jatene in 1975[11], and is known as the *switch operation* or *arterial switch*. This operation involves transection of the great arteries as far distal to their valves as is feasible, excision of the coronary arteries with a generous cuff of aorta, and subsequent anastomosis to their new positions.

Modifications to Jatene's operation include that of Aubert[12], in which an aorticopulmonary septal defect was created, then covered with a patch which included the coronary ostia. The arteries themselves were switched at a second operation.

Yacoub et al.[13] also devised a two-stage correction for simple TGA; this consists of atrial septectomy and banding of the pulmonary artery to allow the left ventricle to develop. This is followed later by arterial switch. Most surgeons seem to prefer the palliative atrial operations of Senning or Mustard for simple transposition, and the switch operation for complex TGA. Successful outcome of either type of operation is dependent upon a number of anatomical variables as well as upon the haemodynamic status of the patient. In either case, the status of the left ventricle is an important factor as the chamber must support the systemic circulation at the completion of the procedure.

The origin and disposition of the coronary arteries have a material bearing on the ease or otherwise of switch procedures, while the presence of additional anomalies, such as pulmonary outflow tract obstruction, influences the choice of operation.

Early death

Atrial operations are low risk procedures: operative mortality is less than 2% [14].

In addition to the complications of cardiopulmonary bypass, *all* patients with TGA are at risk from extensive *myocardial necrosis*. Focal necrosis is a common finding in TGA, irrespective of associated cardiac malformations, and foci of necrosis are almost always to be found after cardiopulmonary bypass, so that the latter is aggravated by the former. In switch operations there is the possibility that a coronary artery may become twisted or kinked, with resulting ischaemia. *Left ventricular failure* in the early postoperative period is sometimes fatal, and a degree of preoperative *right ventricular failure* may progress after operation. *Conduction disturbances* may be due to haemorrhage and/or oedema at the atrioventricular nodal junction following atrial operations. As in most hearts, tedious serial sectioning of the area is seldom necessary, as haemorrhage is usually visible to the naked eye and a few sections from the area will confirm oedema, if this was suspected.

Complications exclusive to atrial operations are:

1. Kinking or compression of the systemic veins.
2. Pulmonary oedema due to too small a new left atrium.
3. Congestive heart failure due to too small a new right atrium.

These are all rare findings at necropsy, as they usually manifest themselves in time for surgical revision.

Complications associated with early death following arterial operations are either concerned with associated malformations (e.g. pulmonary outflow tract obstruction), or with problems arising from the relocation of the coronary arteries. Operative mortality, though greatly reduced in recent years, remains high at 40–60% [15].

Late death

Patients sometimes die suddenly and unexpectedly, months or years after operations for TGA.

The appearance of the heart late after atrial operations is at first sight rather confusing, as the systemic veins seem to pass to the 'wrong' side, and both the size and the morphology of the atria themselves are difficult to recognize. It should be remembered that the atrial operations provide a *pathway* for the respective venous returns only, the chambers as such have been so modified that, in morphological terms, they no longer exist. It follows, then, that a potential finding in late death is either *systemic* or *pulmonary venous obstruction* due to the baffle not having grown with the patient. This is largely a complication of the past, due to improved technique. It is difficult to demonstrate at necropsy because it is very hard to assess the chamber size. If it is difficult to probe the route, either because it is small or because it is tortuous; cautious dissection may reveal a site of obstruction. As this severely damages the specimen, the dissection is best left until the other structures have been evaluated. Pass the probe from the venous end and open with a scalpel or scissors from the arteriovenous valve end.

Poor right *ventricular function* and tricuspid valve regurgitation occur in a significant number of patients: 15% of the former and 9% of the latter[15]. The valve regurgitation is secondary to the poor function, which, in a proportion of cases, developed before the operation. Where myocardial protection was less than optimal at operation, right ventricular dysfunction may develop during operation and manifest much later. Irrespective of function, as in early deaths, focal myocardial necrosis and myocytolysis are anticipated necropsy findings.

Late severe congestive heart failure and dilatation of the right ventricle is an occasional cause of late death in otherwise successful Senning or Mustard repairs.

Serious *arrythmias* have long been held to be a disadvantage of atrial as opposed to switch operations. Mostly these have been overcome by developments in surgical technique so that the coronary sinus and superior cavoatrial junctions are remote from the baffle, but arrythmias occur in TGA patients prior to any operation.

Arrythmias appearing after operation are variously attributed to surgical damage to the sinuatrial node or its artery, or to the atrioventricular node or its artery. As in other conditions (e.g. Fallot's tetralogy), this is unlikely, particularly as they antedate in a number of patients. In the author's experience, fibrosis of the node or bundle has not been a significant necropsy finding.

'Switch' operations

Operative mortality for these operations is mostly associated with ischaemia subsequent to difficulties with relocating the coronary arteries.

Late deaths are likely to be associated with the concurrent cardiac malformations (e.g. VSD) which necessitated a switch operation. In patients with low left ventricular pressure before operation, the status of the morphological (and now functional) left ventricle is crucial to long-term survival. Patients who had a two-stage procedure to prepare the left ventricle had a normal ejection fraction up to 5 years after operation[5], but truly long-term results are as yet unavailable.

The fate of the (often) dilated pulmonary root is as yet unknown in these patients, but in view of the generally deleterious effects of pulmonary valve regurgitation in, for example, Fallot's tetralogy (of which we have nearly 50 years of experience), it is likely to be similar.

References

1. Gittenberger de Groot, A. C., Sauer, U., Oppenheimer-Dekker, A. and Quaegebeur, J. Coronary arterial anatomy in transposition of the great arteries: a morphologic study. *Pediatric Cardiology,* **4** (Supplement 1), 15–24, 1983
2. Sauer, U., Gittenberger de Groot, A. C., Peters, D. R. and Buhlmeyer, K. Cineangiography of the coronary arteries in transposition of the great arteries. *Pediatric Cardiology,* **4** (Supplement 1), 25–42, 1983
3. Blalock, A. and Hanlon, C. R. The surgical treatment of complete transposition of the aorta and pulmonary artery. *Surgery, Gynecology and Obstetrics,* **90,** 1–15, 1950
4. Rashkind, W. J. and Miller, W. M. Creation of an atrial septal defect without thoracotomy: a palliative approach to complete transposition of the great arteries. *Journal of the American Medical Association,* **196,** 991–992, 1966
5. Mustard, W. T., Chute, A. L., Keith, J. D. *et al.* A surgical approach to transposition of the great vessels with extracorporeal circuit. *Surgery,* **36,** 39–51, 1954

6. Baffes, T. G. A new method for surgical correction for transposition of the aorta and pulmonary artery. *Surgery, Gynecology and Obstetrics,* **102**, 227–233, 1954
7. Senning, A. Surgical correction of transposition of the great vessels. *Surgery,* **45**, 966–980, 1959
8. Mustard, W. T. Successful two-stage correction of transposition of the great vessels. *Surgery,* **55**, 469–472, 1964
9. Rastelli, G. C., McGoon, D. C. and Wallace, R. B. Anatomic correction of transposition of the great arteries with ventricular septal defect and subpulmonary stenosis. *Journal of Thoracic and Cardiovascular Surgery,* **58**, 545–552, 1969
10. McGoon, D. C. Intraventricular repair of transposition of the great arteries. *Journal of Thoracic and Cardiovascular Surgery,* **64**, 430–434, 1972
11. Jatene, A. D., Fontes, V. F., Paulista, P. P. *et al.* Anatomic correction of transposition of the great vessels. *Journal of Thoracic and Cardiovascular Surgery,* **73**, 363–370, 1976
12. Aubert, J., Pannetier, A., Courvelly, J. P. *et al.* Transposition of the great arteries: new technique for anatomical correction. *British Heart Journal,* **40**, 204–208, 1978
13. Yacoub, M. H., Radley-Smith, R. and MacLaurin, R. Two-stage operation for anatomical correction of transposition of the great arteries with intact ventricular septum. *Lancet,* **i**, 1275–1278, 1977
14. Williams, W. G., Freedom, R. M., Duncan, W. J. *et al.* Indications for arterial repair of complete transposition of the great arteries. *Pediatric Cardiology,* **4** (Supplement 1), 93–98, 1983
15. Williams, W. G., Trusler, G. A., Freedom, F. W. *et al.* Results of arterial repair of transposition: the Toronto experience. *Pediatric Cardiology,* **4** (Supplement 1), 99–104, 1983

Index